Introducing Nicotinamide Mononucleotide (NMN): Optimising Health and Beyond

Exploring NMN through human clinical trials and the potential nutrients and herbs that may enhance its potential

Brad McEwen PhD, MHSc (HumNut), MPH

Vitamedicine Institute

First Edition – Published 2025

Vitamedicine Institute
Warriewood, NSW, Australia

ISBN: 978-0-646-72614-4 (sc)

CONTENTS

About the Author

Dr Brad McEwen PhD is a distinguished expert in preventive and personalised health, with a particular focus on optimising longevity and healthspan, and enhancing cardiometabolic, mental, and cognitive health and wellbeing. Over a career spanning more than 26 years, he has established himself as a highly respected naturopath, nutritionist, herbalist, educator, researcher, and mentor.

Dr Brad holds a PhD from the University of Sydney, as well as a Master of Health Science (Human Nutrition) and a Master of Public Health from Deakin University. He is also formally qualified in naturopathy, nutrition, herbal medicine, and sports medicine. This multidisciplinary background underpins his integrated approach to advancing individual and population health.

Throughout his career, Dr Brad has contributed extensively to higher education and professional development in health and complementary medicine. He has delivered seminars, webinars, and conference presentations both nationally and internationally, including in France, the United States, the United Kingdom, Spain, Japan, and New Zealand. He has served on an academic board, various academic and research committees, and course advisory committees, and continues to act as a peer reviewer for international scientific journals.

Dr Brad's research explores the influence of diet, nutrition, and lifestyle medicine on longevity, healthspan, and a wide range of conditions, including cardiovascular disease, cardiometabolic syndrome, depression, anxiety, cognitive health, stress, polycystic ovary syndrome, chronic fatigue syndrome, and other chronic diseases. His work is published regularly in peer-reviewed journals and reflects a strong commitment to evidence-based practice.

Beyond his research and academic contributions, Dr Brad is engaged in public health advocacy. He is committed to expanding access to health services, promoting chronic disease prevention, improving the availability of nutritious food and health education within schools, and championing health equity. He played a pivotal role in developing a Bachelor of Health Science (Honours) degree and currently serves on the Board of Directors of the Australian Traditional-Medicine Society (ATMS), the nation's largest professional association for natural medicine practitioners.

In his current role as Head of Products and Innovation at a leading health manufacturing company, Dr Brad oversees the development of innovative health products, ensuring scientific rigour and regulatory compliance.

Dr Brad's contributions have been recognised with numerous national and international awards, including the Complementary Medicines Australia Industry Contributor of the Year Award (which honours and recognises the consistent, dedicated contribution of an individual or team to the advancement and promotion of the complementary medicine industry), the prestigious Eberhard F. Mammen Young Investigator Award (an international award recognising contributions in the field of thrombosis and haemostasis), the Excellence in Practice Lecturer Researcher of the Year Award, and the Dorothy Hall Memorial Award for Practitioner Excellence (which acknowledges his contributions to advancing natural medicine in Australia). He has also been a multiple-time finalist for Practitioner of the Year, Researcher of the Year, and Educator/Lecturer of the Year.

Regularly sought after for his insights, Dr Brad has featured in podcasts, radio, and print media. He remains actively engaged in ongoing professional education and is passionate about supporting others to achieve their potential. Outside of his professional life, he enjoys travel, photography, walking, good conversation, and the occasional piece of chocolate.

Dr Brad McEwen

PhD, MHSc (HumNut), MPH, GradCertHSc (HumNut), BHSc, AdvDipNat, DBM, DNut, DSM, DRM, Fellow ATMS

Instagram: bradmcewenphd

YouTube: drbradmcewenphd

LinkedIn: bradmcewen

Acknowledgements

I consider myself fortunate to have been surrounded by exceptional people throughout my life. I have always been someone who preferred to offer help rather than ask for it. Seeing others achieve their dreams and exceed their goals brings me great joy and happiness. Although I'm hesitant to ask for assistance, I've found that in moments when I needed encouragement or support, the right people appeared, and circumstances fell into place.

For my Mum, my sister Samantha, nephew Patrick, Uncle Garey and Aunty Kerrie, and my cousins Natalee and Carlton – thank you all for your love and support.

I am deeply grateful to express my heartfelt appreciation and recognition to the people who have been a constant source of inspiration, unwavering support, encouragement, and unwavering belief in both myself and my passions: Thomas Azimi, Lola Berry, Dr Jeffrey Bland, Professor Kerry Bone, Professor Lesley Braun, Lucy Canny, Jenna Carroll, Craig Fallshaw, Kiri Fleming, Professor Sandra Grace, Georgia Hartmann, Dr Jason Hawrelak, Dr Leah Hechtman, Bob Kent, Leisa Macnamara, Lincoln Macnamara, Tegan Martin, Sally Panton, Anna Robards, Jessica Sepel, Justin Sinclair, Professor Geoffrey Tofler, Professor Christopher Ward, Professor Jon Wardle, Smit Zaveri, and the team at Complementary Medicines Group.

I would love to acknowledge the countless friends, colleagues, students, practitioners, researchers, and educators who consistently motivate and inspire me. I am truly blessed to know and be connected with such amazing people. Thank you all.

Introduction

I first started teaching about the functions of nicotinamide mononucleotide (NMN) to college students in 2004. I was interested in the functions of NMN and NAD in the body and their potential benefits for extending lifespan and increasing longevity.

Health represents a harmonious state of balance, an equilibrium that an individual has established within oneself (internally) and between oneself and their social and physical environment (externally).[1] The state of an individual's health is determined by their ability to maintain a sense of balance within themselves and with the world around them.

Optimum nutrition is the foundation of health. Vitamins, minerals, and other nutrients may be chosen and utilised for their antidepressant,[2] anti-inflammatory,[3-7] antioxidant,[8-10] anti-anxiety (anxiolytic),[2] bone health,[11,12] brain signalling,[13] cell function,[14,15] DNA metabolism,[8,16] energy metabolism.[17,18] glucose metabolism,[19,20] immune system health,[21] among other functions. Herbal medicines support health and wellbeing and have been used for thousands of years for the prevention and management of various health conditions, particularly chronic disease.[22-24] Herbs may be chosen and utilised for their adaptogen,[25] anti-inflammatory,[26-29] antioxidant,[27-30] anxiolytic,[31-33] hepatoprotective,[34-36] immunomodulatory,[27-29] nerve tonic,[37,38] among other properties.

NMN is a precursor of nicotinamide adenine dinucleotide (NAD^+).[39] NAD^+ and the NAD^+-derived cofactors (NADH, $NADP^+$, NADPH) are essential for cellular energy metabolism, homeostasis and growth.[39] Some of the functions of NMN include increasing NAD^+

levels,[40-46] increasing cellular energy,[47] improving mitochondrial bioenergetics,[44] energy metabolism,[43] anti-inflammatory,[41,42,48] antioxidant,[42,43] reducing reactive oxygen species (ROS),[41,43,49] reducing oxidative stress,[41,42] activating SIRT1,[42,50] improving mitochondrial dynamics[44] and function,[40,49] and having potential anti-ageing effects.[42]

Although extensive in-vitro and preclinical research has been conducted on NMN (see Part 2), this book focuses on the various functions of NMN supported by the findings from human clinical trials.

Introducing Nicotinamide Mononucleotide (NMN): Optimising Health and Beyond is structured in three main parts to guide readers through the science and application of NMN. Part 1 introduces the foundations of health, longevity, and healthy ageing, with an overview of key processes such as mitochondrial function, telomeres and telomerase, inflammation, and oxidative stress. Part 2 introduces NMN and its role in the body, along with findings from human clinical trials, and the daily doses used in research. Part 3 explores a range of vitamins, minerals, nutrients, and herbs that may be taken alongside NMN or considered in combination when formulating products, offering a broader perspective on supporting health and wellbeing.

PART 1. Optimising Health

What is Health?

What is health, and what is optimised health? Health is central to human development. Health can be seen as an indicator and an outcome of progress in sustainable development.[51] The World Health Organization (WHO) has defined health as "a state of complete physical, mental and social well-being and not merely the absence of disease or infirmity".[52] Another definition of health is that health is a state of balance, an equilibrium that an individual has established within oneself and between oneself and their social and physical environment.[1]

Health is associated with optimal health and the access to health care and education.[53] Health represents a harmonious state of balance, an equilibrium that an individual has established within oneself (internally) and between oneself and their social and physical environment (externally).[1] The state of an individual's health is determined by their ability to maintain a sense of balance within themselves and with the world around them, homeostasis. Homeostasis serves as the fundamental unifying principle in the field of physiology, characterised as a self-regulating mechanism through which an organism maintains internal equilibrium while adapting to changing and fluctuating external environments.[54] Health is the ability to adapt to one's environment.[55] Health is not a fixed entity. The capacity and ability for adaptation allow us to maintain flexibility in the face of evolving influences and dynamic forces that affect and determine the health and wellbeing of individuals and communities alike. Adaptability empowers accredited health practitioners to address health issues by taking into account the unique circumstances and contextual factors relevant to specific conditions at a given time and location.[55]

The Ottawa Charter for Health Promotion (1986) notes that health promotion is the process of enabling people to increase control over their health and being able to improve their health.[56] In order to achieve a state of holistic wellness encompassing physical, mental, emotional, and social aspects, it is imperative for an individual to possess the ability to recognise and achieve personal aspirations, ambitions, and objectives, to fulfill essential needs, and adapt or manage their surroundings. Health is perceived as a valuable asset that enhances daily existence, extending beyond mere survival.[56] Think of it as thriving in all areas, not just surviving. Health is a positive concept emphasising social and personal resources, as well as physical capacities.[56] The enjoyment of the highest attainable standard of health is one of the fundamental rights of every human.[52] Optimised health is essential to everyone.

Suboptimal health status refers to a general physical condition that exists on a continuum between health and illness. It is characterised by the experience of health-related complaints, persistent fatigue, and a range of physical symptoms affecting various systems, including the cardiovascular, digestive, and immune systems, as well as mental health. This condition typically persists for a minimum duration of three months.[57] The history and progression of a disease can be categorised into several stages: the underlying stage, the susceptible stage, the subclinical stage, the clinical stage, and the final outcomes of recovery, disability, or death.[57] Research indicates that most people do not seek care until a disease process has already manifested, where they notice clear and unmistakable symptoms of a disease.[58] By postponing care, individuals may miss critical opportunities for treatment that could improve their health outcomes and overall quality of life.[58]

A brief look at Longevity, Healthspan, and Healthy Ageing

In recent decades, there have been significant advances and increases in human longevity.[59] In this section, I'll briefly discuss longevity, healthspan, and healthy ageing. Lifespan is the total number of years lived by an individual.[60] At the turn of the 20th century, life expectancy at birth in most of today's developed nations ranged between 45 and 50 years, with women routinely outliving men.[61] Life expectancy has increased by three decades since the mid-twentieth century.[60] From 1950 to 2020, the average life expectancy, a benchmark of population health, has risen from 47 to 73 years of age.[60] This equates to a 26-year expansion in these seven decades.[60] The world population continues to grow.[60] In many countries, the average life expectancy currently exceeds 80 years of age.[59] The number of countries with more than one-fifth of their population composed of those over 70 years of age continues to grow.[60] The World Health Organization (WHO) predicts that by 2030, people over 60 years of age will outnumber children younger than 10 years of age, and by 2050 the over-60 population will number 2.1 billion.[62] Although this increase of lifespan has been seen as a positive advancement, it has come at a cost. This cost is an increase in age-related diseases.[59] Age-related and chronic diseases include neurological disorders,[59] cardiovascular diseases,[59,63] type 2 diabetes,[59,63] stroke,[63] kidney disease,[63] pulmonary diseases,[63] musculoskeletal disorders,[59] and some cancers.[59,63]

Healthspan is the number of years lived in good health and disease-free,[60,64,65] or free from age-related diseases[66,67] and disabilities of ageing,[67] until the onset of such diseases, leading to a period of morbidity.[66] In short, healthspan is the functional and disease-free period of life.[65] This definition of healthspan enables us to view healthspan as a measurable and quantitative continuous parameter, similar to how we view lifespan.[67] Prolonging the healthspan ultimately leads to an extension of the overall lifespan.[66] The concept of healthspan emphasises quality of life.[64]

There is a recognised gap between lifespan, i.e., the total life lived, and healthspan, i.e., the period free from disease. The healthspan-lifespan gap is estimated to be approximately nine years when assessed through health-adjusted life expectancy, which takes into account factors such as overall life expectancy, the duration of life lived with disabilities, and the impact of premature mortality due to disease.[60] Extending lifespan alone without delaying disease onset and/or reducing disease severity would actually aggravate the healthspan-lifespan gap.[60] See Figure 1 for examples of lifespan vs healthspan. A guiding principle in addressing the healthspan-lifespan gap is in achieving health as "a state of complete physical, mental and social well-being and not merely the absence of disease or infirmity" per the World Health Organization (WHO).[52]

The concept of healthy ageing encompasses an ongoing continuing process to enhance and maintain physical and mental wellbeing, autonomy, independence, and overall quality of life across an individual's lifespan.[68] Healthy ageing is adding healthy years to life by promoting health and wellbeing, rather than solely focusing on increasing chronological age and extending the number of years lived.[69] Maintaining a high standard of "living" is essential for the overall health, quality of life, and happiness of older individuals. It goes beyond simply being free from illness, encompassing aspects such as finding purpose and meaning in life, nurturing connections with others, experiencing wellbeing despite health challenges, and retaining physical and mental health and independence.[68] If a person ages unhealthily, it could be seen as expanding the morbidity span.[66]

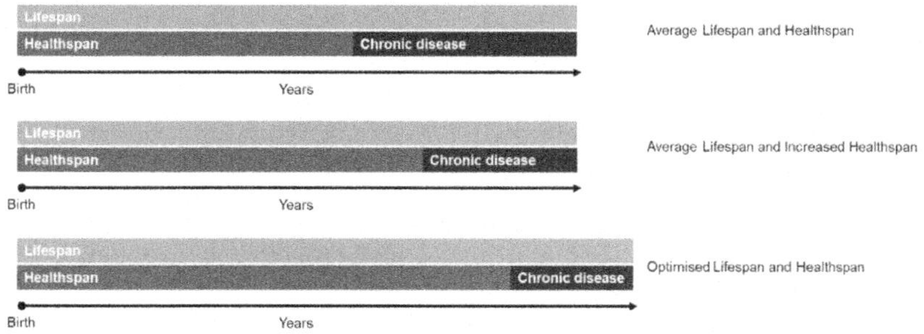

Figure 1. Examples of Lifespan vs Healthspan

Ageing is characterised as the gradual and progressive impairment and dysfunction of molecular and cellular processes, leading to reduced physiological function and heightened vulnerability to diseases.[70] A key feature of the ageing process is mitochondrial dysfunction, which correlates with elevated oxidative stress and diminished antimicrobial defences.[70] Genomic instability appears to be a fundamental factor in the ageing process, and the accumulation of DNA damage plays a substantial role in various early senility disorders.[71] As we age, telomeres become shorter, resulting in telomere attrition and a heightened susceptibility to diseases associated with tissue regeneration.[71] Ageing is intimately linked with metabolism.[72]

The twelve hallmarks of ageing[73] are:

- genomic instability
- telomere attrition
- epigenetic alterations
- loss of proteostasis
- disabled macroautophagy
- deregulated nutrient-sensing
- mitochondrial dysfunction
- cellular senescence
- stem cell exhaustion
- altered intercellular communication
- chronic inflammation
- dysbiosis

A brief look at the mitochondria

A brief look into the mighty mitochondria. Due to all of the known functions and potential functions of the mitochondria, I could write a whole book on the mitochondria, so I will try to keep this very brief…

Mitochondria consist of unique outer and inner membranes that enclose the intermembrane space and matrix compartments.[74] Mitochondria are unique and distinctive organelles because, unlike other cellular components, they possess their own genome, which is made up of mitochondrial DNA (mtDNA).[74,75]

Mitochondria are often called the powerhouses of the cell.[76] Mitochondria are the primary site of cellular energy production (bioenergetics).[75,76] The inner mitochondrial membrane encloses a central compartment termed the matrix.[75] The energy currency of cells, produced by mitochondria, is evident in the synthesis of the high-energy phosphate molecule adenosine-5'-triphosphate (ATP), through a mechanism known as oxidative phosphorylation.[74,75] Within the mitochondrial matrix, enzymes of the tricarboxylic acid cycle produce electron carriers (NADH and $FADH_2$), which subsequently transfer electrons to the electron transport chain located in the inner membrane.[74] The proton gradient generated by complexes I, III, and IV is discharged via the rotary turbine-like ATP synthase apparatus, also known as complex V, which facilitates the phosphorylation of ADP into ATP.[74] Sirtuin proteins represent a highly conserved family of proteins.[76] SIRT3 functions as a deacetylase enzyme situated within the mitochondria and plays a crucial role in energy metabolism.[76] The majority of proteins that participate in energy metabolism are modulated through acetylation and deacetylation processes, with SIRT3 serving as the primary deacetylase protein in the mitochondria.[76] SIRT1 plays an important role in maintaining a balance between mitochondrial biogenesis and degradation by mitophagy.[76] An elevated demand for ATP is addressed by augmenting mitochondrial mass and stimulating oxidative phosphorylation. For instance, a rise in mitochondrial mass and function is noted following endurance training. The control of mitochondrial biogenesis is closely linked with mechanisms that promote vascularisation, improve oxygen transport to tissues, and support oxygen availability to enable the effective mitochondrial oxidation of glucose and fatty acids.[74] Mitochondria contribute to fatty acid and amino acid metabolism.[75]

Mitochondria are vital for maintaining cellular and organismal homeostasis through the integral role they play in cellular bioenergetics,[75] metabolic precursor synthesis,[75] calcium regulation,[75] ROS production,[75] immune signalling,[75] and apoptosis.[75]

Mitochondrial reactive oxygen species (ROS) play a significant and vital role in influencing and modulating homeostatic signalling pathways, which are essential for regulating cell proliferation and differentiation.[74] Mitochondria contribute to cell signalling and function as a reservoir of critical second messengers[75] and effector molecules,[75] such as damage-associated molecular patterns (DAMPs),[75] inflammasomes,[75] and sirtuins,[75] that mediate essential cellular and physiological processes.[75] Additionally, mitochondria contribute to adaptive stress signalling pathways, including those activated by hypoxia.[74]

Mitochondria play a vital role in maintaining cellular homeostasis by regulating intracellular Ca^{2+} concentrations through the processes of uptake,[75] storage,[75,76] and release of Ca^{2+},[75] and can regulate calcium responses.[76] In neurons, the capacity of mitochondria to regulate Ca^{2+} flux is crucial for the management of neurotransmitter release, neurogenesis, and neuronal plasticity.[74] Mitochondria provide substantial amounts of ATP along with tricarboxylic acid (TCA) cycle intermediates, which act as essential components for the synthesis of the neurotransmitters GABA and glutamate. Mitochondrial function and behaviour are central to the physiology of humans.[74] Mitochondria play a crucial role in the biosynthesis of haem.[75] Mitochondria mediate cell proliferation, differentiation and death.[76] Mitochondrial diseases can affect any organ system and manifest at any age.[74] Mitochondrial dysfunction has been implicated in a wide range of diseases,[74] such as neurological disorders,[76]

Mitochondrial dysfunction is associated with ageing[77] and represents a significant hallmark of ageing.[78,79] Mitochondrial dysfunction, which is operationally characterised by a reduced respiratory capacity per mitochondrion along with a diminished mitochondrial membrane potential, is usually associated with an elevated production of oxygen free radicals (e.g., ROS).[79] This condition serves both as a cause and a consequence of cellular senescence and plays a significant role in various feedback loops that initiate and sustain the senescent phenotype.[79]

Mitochondrial dysfunction is closely connected to the decline in skeletal muscle associated with advancing age.[78] Research indicates that compromised mitochondrial function correlates with reduced walking speed, increased muscle fatigue, diminished strength, and, ultimately, the onset of sarcopenia.[78] Consequently, enhancing mitochondrial health emerges as a promising approach to strengthen muscle health.

A brief look at telomeres and telomerase

Within the nucleus of all cells, DNA chains are tightly coiled into chromosomes.[80] Telomeres are repetitive DNA segments (protein-DNA complexes) that form protective caps at the ends of the chromosomes.[80-

[83] Think of the aglet (plastic) at the end of a shoelace. The aglet holds the shoelace together and stops it from fraying. Telomere caps chromosome ends and protects them from being recognised and processed as DNA breaks.[83] These telomeres are structures that protect the genetic material of the cell and keep the DNA chains from unravelling, sticking to one another, or fraying.[80] Telomeres are essential for chromosome stability.[84] The loss of the capping function of telomeres results in genetic instability,[83,85] loss of cellular viability,[83] cell growth arrest,[85] and cell death.[85] Each time a cell divides, the chromosomes are replicated, and with each replication, the telomeres are shortened slightly.[80] In essence, during cellular division, the telomere is not entirely replicated due to the constraints of DNA polymerases in completing the replication of the ends of linear DNA molecules, resulting in telomere shortening with each replication.[86] The average cell loses from 30 to 200 base pairs from the end of the telomere with each division. As cell division continues, the telomeres then become progressively shorter. Eventually, this can lead to cellular senescence or death.[80]

Telomeric DNA is composed of tandemly repeated, frequently short, sequence motifs that generally include clusters of three or four guanines (for instance, TTAGGG (T_2AG_3) in humans).[81,83,85,86] These telomeric repeats are synthesised by the enzyme telomerase, which is a ribonucleoprotein complex made up of a reverse transcriptase-like subunit (TERT) and a substantial RNA subunit (TER) that provides the template for the telomeric DNA repeat. The G-rich strand elongates in the 3’ direction, resulting in a single-stranded overhang that serves as the substrate for the elongation mediated by telomerase.[83] Recent findings indicate that telomeres are present in at least two distinct configurations or states: an 'open' complex and a 'closed' complex. The 'closed' complex is believed to signify the condition that caps and safeguards the ends of chromosomes.[83]

Telomere length is regulated by the enzyme telomerase and is linked to exposure to proinflammatory cytokines and oxidative stress.[87] Telomerase is the enzyme that helps rebuild and extend the telomeres of chromosomes by adding base pairs. Telomeres and telomerase, as protectors of cellular DNA, play important roles in health and disease.[80] Telomerase is important for telomere formation, maintenance, and restoration. [87] Telomerase has direct telomere-protective functions.[86]

The ageing process is linked to telomere shortening.[80] Telomere length can serve as a biomarker of a cell's biological age, versus chronological age.[86] Shorter telomeres have been associated with maladaptive cellular changes,[88] blocked cell division,[88] interference with tissue replenishment,[88] age-related diseases,[87] and early mortality.[87] The cellular environment significantly influences the regulation of telomere length and the activity of telomerase. Oxidative stress has the potential to reduce telomere length, while antioxidants may help to slow down this shortening.[86]

A very brief look at inflammation and oxidative stress

Inflammation means "to set on fire".[89] Inflammation is the immune system's response to harmful stimuli, such as damaged cells, toxic compounds, pathogens, or radiation. Inflammation acts by removing damaging stimuli and initiating the healing process.[90] Inflammation and the dysregulation of inflammatory pathways lead to the development of chronic diseases,[89] including neurodegenerative diseases,[89] neurological diseases,[89] respiratory diseases,[89] cardiovascular diseases,[89,90] atherosclerosis,[90] type 2 diabetes,[89] asthma,[90] autoimmune diseases,[90] arthritis,[89,90] cancer,[89,90] non-alcoholic fatty liver disease,[91] and bowel diseases.[90]

Oxidative stress occurs from the imbalance between the body's antioxidant defences and reactive oxygen species (ROS) and reactive nitrogen species (RNS) production.[92] Oxidative stress and free radical damage are involved in the initiation and progression of numerous chronic conditions, such as cognitive conditions,[92] neurodegenerative diseases,[92] cardiovascular diseases,[90,92] hypertension,[90] atherosclerosis,[90] type 2 diabetes,[90,92] chronic kidney disease,[92] chronic obstructive pulmonary disease (COPD),[92] asthma,[90] non-alcoholic fatty liver disease (NAFLD),[91] autoimmune diseases,[90] macular degeneration,[92] cancer,[90,92] sarcopenia,[92] and frailty.[92]

PART 2. NICOTINAMIDE MONONUCLEOTIDE (NMN)

Firstly, what is NAD^+?

Firstly, what is NAD^+? Nicotinamide adenine dinucleotide (NAD) is a multifunctional molecule found in all living cells.[93] It is critical for life.[94] NAD^+ (the oxidised form of NAD)[95,96] It is one of the most abundant molecules in the human body, at approximately three grams in the average person.[95] NAD^+ is extensively compartmentalised within the cellular environment.[94] The concentrations of both total and free NAD^+ are elevated in the mitochondria compared to the cytosol, and mitochondrial NAD can be maintained even in situations that reduce total tissue concentrations.[94] NAD^+ undergoes continuous processes of synthesis, degradation, and recycling, occurring not only in the cytoplasm but also within key organelles such as the nucleus, Golgi apparatus, and peroxisomes.[95] NAD^+ levels decline with age.[95] NAD^+ is found in serum and the extracellular environment, and some evidence indicates that NMN may also be present in these areas.[95] Circulating precursors of NAD^+ could play a role in coordinating NAD^+ biosynthesis and facilitating communication between different organs.[95]

NAD is essential for life.[94,97] It is a signalling molecule that determines and directs the health and lifespan of eukaryotes.[97] NAD is a vital metabolic redox co-enzyme that is necessary for over 500 enzymatic reactions.[95,98] NAD^+ has numerous functions, such as:

- Participating in many metabolic reactions[94,99]
- Metabolism[98]
- Modulating metabolic signalling pathways[93]
- DNA repair[95,98,100]
- DNA damage response[96]
- Gene expression[93,98]
- Transcription[96,99]
- Cell division[95]
- Epigenetic regulation[100]
- Mitochondrial function[43,95,98]
- Stimulate cell survival[47]
- Redox reactions[95,96,98,100]
- Cell function[95]
- Signalling[100]
- Protein-protein signalling[95]
- Regulation of calcium homeostasis[43,93]
- Co-substrate for the addition of poly-ADP-ribose to proteins[98]
- Poly-ADP ribose and poly-ADP-ribose polymerases (PARPs)[94,98]
- Essential substrate for sirtuins[94,101]
- Sirtuin activation[96]
- Energy metabolism[43,100]
- Aerobic energy metabolic reactions[43]
- Maintenance of myocardial bioenergetic efficiency[100]

- Acting as a cofactor in the breakdown of glucose and fat[72]
- Glycolysis[96]
- Tricarboxylic acid cycle (Kreb's cycle) activity[96]
- Mitochondrial respiration[96]
- Fatty acid beta-oxidation[96,100]
- Immune response[95]
- Anti-inflammation[98]
- Plays a vital role in energy metabolism in important reproductive (e.g., folliculogenesis, oocyte maturation, and ovulation)[41]

NAD^+ is critical for human health and longevity,[98,99] ageing,[93,98,101] circadian rhythm,[95] cell survival,[98] along with aspects of degeneration[93] and cell death.[93,98] NAD^+ affects longevity and transcriptional silencing through the regulation of the Sir2p family, which are NAD-dependent deacetylases.[99] A deficiency of NAD^+ is significantly associated with a range of pathophysiological conditions, such as type 2 diabetes, heart failure, obesity, Alzheimer's disease, and cerebral ischaemia.[98] As individuals age, the levels of NAD^+ decrease in multiple organs, which plays a role in the onset of numerous age-related diseases.[98] The declining NAD^+ levels is associated with lower energy production, compromised genomic signalling, and DNA repair mechanisms.[96]

Biosynthesis of NAD^+

NAD^+ levels are controlled by balancing biosynthesis and salvage on one side, and breakdown on the other side.[72] NAD^+ can be synthesised from the amino acid tryptophan,[47,72,94-96] and via its prime precursors nicotinamide,[47,72,94-96,100,102] nicotinic acid,[47,72,94-96,100] nicotinamide riboside (NR),[47,72,95,96,100] and nicotinamide mononucleotide (NMN)[47,72,95,96,100,102] (Figure 2) NAD^+ is primarily synthesised through NMN.[98] NMN is one of the last steps in the NAD^+ synthesis.[96] There are several different NAD^+ biosynthesis pathways: the Preiss-Handler, in which NAD is synthesised from nicotinic acid[47];[98] de novo synthesis, which starts from tryptophan;[47,95,98] and the salvage pathway.[47,95,98]

In the Preiss-Handler pathway, nicotinic acid is transported into the cell by either SLC5A8 or SLC22A13 transporter.[96] The Preiss-Handler pathway initiates with the conversion of nicotinic acid into nicotinic acid mononucleotide (NAMN) through the action of the enzyme nicotinic acid phosphoribosyltransferase (NAPRT). Subsequently, NAMN is utilised in the biosynthesis of nicotinic acid adenine dinucleotide ($NAAD^+$) by nicotinamide/nicotinic acid mononucleotide adenylyltransferase (NMNAT1/2/3).[96,98] Ultimately, NAD^+ synthetase (NADS) converts $NAAD^+$ into NAD^+ with the involvement of ammonia and ATP as additional components.[98]

In the de novo pathway, tryptophan is transported into the cell by transporters SLC7A5 and SLC36A4.[96] The de novo synthesis pathway for NAD^+ consists of eight steps, commencing with indoleamine 2,3-dioxygenase (IDO) or tryptophan 2,3-dioxygenase (TDO), which catalyse the conversion of tryptophan into N-formylkynurenine.[98] Subsequently, N-formylkynurenine undergoes transformation into kynurenine through the action of formamidase (KFase). Following this, kynurenine 3-hydroxylase (K3H) introduces a hydroxyl group, resulting in the formation of 3-hydroxy-kynurenine.[98] This compound is then converted into 3-hydroxyanthranilate, which is further processed into 2-

amino-3-carboxymuconate semialdehyde (ACMS) via the enzymes kynureninase (Kyase) and 3-hydroxyanthranilate-3,4-dioxygenase. 2-amino-3-carboxymuconate semialdehyde subsequently cyclises to yield quinolinic acid (QA), which plays a role in the biosynthesis of NAMN in conjunction with quinolinate phosphoribosyltransferase (QPRT). The final two steps mirror those of the Preiss-Handler pathway, wherein NAD^+ is synthesised sequentially from NAMN and NAAD through the actions of NMNAT 1/2/3 and NADS.[98]

The salvage pathway serves as the main source of NAD^+ in mammalian cells.[96,98] The breakdown of NAD^+ and the subsequent production of nicotinamide (as a by-product) are facilitated by NAD-consuming enzymes, including sirtuins,[72,95,98] poly(ADP-ribose) polymerases (PARPs),[72,95,96,98] glycohydrolase CD38,[95,98] nucleotide phosphatase CD73,[95] glycohydrolase CD157,[95,98] cyclic ADP-ribose synthases,[72] and toll/interleukin-1 receptor (TIR) domain of sterile alpha and TIR motif-containing protein 1 (SARM1).[95,98] This pathway consists of only two steps. The synthesis rate of NAD^+ within this pathway is primarily regulated by NAMPT, which transforms nicotinamide and 5-phosphoribosyl-1-pyrophosphate (PRPP) into NMN during the first step.[98] Subsequently, NMN, which acts as the substrate for NAMNT, is linked to ATP and converted into NAD in the second step.[98] PARPs and cyclic ADP-ribose synthases are especially important in maintaining NAD^+ balance.[72] Under normal conditions, the activity of NAMPT is preserved to maintain NAD^+ homeostasis. The activity of NAMPT declines with advancing age and is further exacerbated by health conditions such as acute lung injury, atherosclerosis, cancer, type 2 diabetes, rheumatoid arthritis, and sepsis.[95]

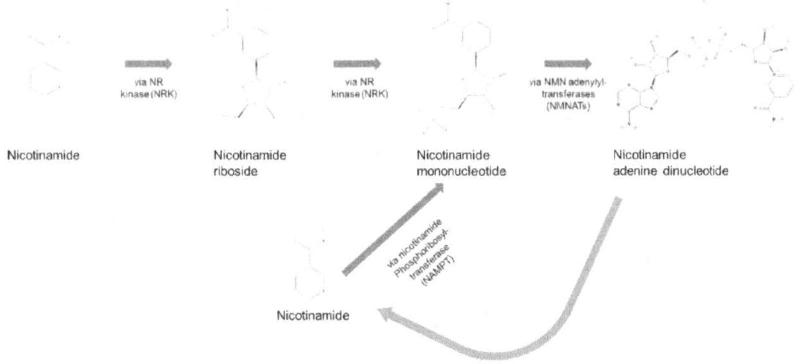

Figure 2. Nicotinamide adenine dinucleotide (NAD) biosynthesis[95,98,102-106]

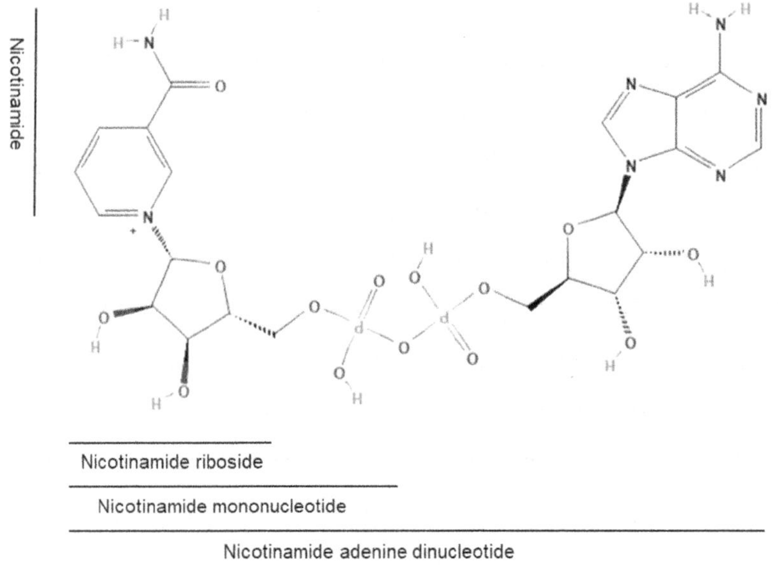

Figure 3. Nicotinamide adenine dinucleotide (NAD) biosynthesis visualisation[106] (adapted from[100])

Ageing and NAD+ levels

Ageing and age-associated conditions are attributed to decreasing levels of NAD^+.[96] NAD^+ availability decreases with age and in certain disease conditions.[46] Ageing represents a gradual physiological transformation within an organism that culminates in senescence, characterised by a reduction in energy production within the mitochondria of various tissues, including the brain, skin, pancreas, skeletal muscle, adipose tissue, and liver. This decline is partly attributed to a decrease in NAD^+ levels and a reduced ability and capacity of the organism to adapt to metabolic stress.[71] The reduction in NAD^+ levels, associated with inflammation, exacerbates oxidative stress and disrupts normal cellular function, resulting in increased apoptosis and a notable decrease in oocyte quality.[41]

The amount of NAD^+ in the body decreases as people age.[46,94,96] The reduction in NAD^+ levels is primarily due to its utilisation by enzymes such as poly (ADP-ribose) polymerase (PARPs),[71,94,96] due to DNA damage,[94] NADase (CD38/CD157),[71,94] CD38 (due to inflammation),[94] NAD^+-dependent acetylase (sirtuins),[71] sterile alpha and TIR motif (SARM),[94] tankyrase (TNKS),[71] and bone marrow stromal cell antigen 1 (BST1).[71] Among these enzymes, CD38 is particularly significant as it may contribute to the reduction of NAD^+ associated with the ageing process.[71] Enzymes that consume NAD^+ play a pivotal role in regulating numerous cellular processes, including mitochondrial protection, stem cell rejuvenation, and DNA repair, all of which are vital for sustaining cellular health. Nevertheless, these processes ultimately lead to a significant depletion of NAD^+.[71] However, the administration of NMN can help restore the balance of NAD^+ biosynthesis.[71]

The reduction in systemic NAD^+ biosynthesis may serve as a crucial catalyst for numerous pathophysiological alterations that substantially influence the ageing process by diminishing the functions of SIRT1 and other sirtuins.[72] NAD^+ is essential for the activation of sirtuins.[96] Sirtuins are essential in the regulation of various cellular functions, including cell growth,[98] energy metabolism,[98] stress resistance,[96,98] inflammation,[98] and the functioning of neuronal circadian rhythms,[98] among other roles.[98] Sirtuins are linked to positive effects in anti-aging and longevity.[96]

SIRT1 is expressed throughout numerous tissues and engages with proteins found in both the nucleus and the cytosol.[39] The level of NAD+ within the cell directly influences the enzymatic activity of SIRT1 as well as its regulatory roles.[39] Sirtuins employ NAD^+ to execute a wide range of functions, including deacetylase, lipoamidase, deglutarylase, desuccinylase, and demalonylase activities. The expression of sirtuins is closely associated with ageing, lifespan extension, and age-related physiological alterations. CD38 utilises NAD^+ to generate nicotinamide and ADP-ribose, while PARP employs NAD^+ to synthesise branched ADP-ribose polymers that are essential for DNA repair.[71] Reduced NAD^+ levels have been linked to all the hallmarks of ageing.[96] The declining NAD^+ levels are associated with lower energy production, compromised genomic signalling, and DNA repair mechanisms.[96] Ageing-related inflammation and oxidative stress have been demonstrated to impair the NAMPT-mediated biosynthesis of NAD^+.[98] The progression of chronic inflammation associated with ageing may play a role in the suppression of NAMPT-mediated NAD^+ biosynthesis as well as the CLOCK/BMAL-mediated circadian mechanisms.[98]

What is NMN?

Nicotinamide mononucleotide (NMN) is a water-soluble[107] bioactive nucleotide formed by the reaction between a nucleoside containing ribose, nicotinamide (NAM), and a phosphate group.[47,98,107,108] Nicotinamide is directly converted to NMN through the action of nicotinamide phosphoribosyl transferase (NAMPT).[71,98] NAMPT serves as a rate-limiting enzyme in the synthesis of NAD^+, which is present in both intracellular and extracellular forms, referred to as iNAMPT and eNAMPT, respectively.[71]

The molecular formula of NMN is $C_{11}H_{15}N_2O_8P$[42,105,107] and its molecular weight is 334.22 g/mol.[105,107] There are two anomeric forms of NMN, namely alpha (α-) and beta (β-).[42,47,98] The beta (β-) anomer is the active form.[42,47,98]

NMN is one of the intermediates in nicotinamide adenine dinucleotide (NAD^+) biosynthesis.[47,98] It can be described as a potent precursor for NAD^+. Blood NAD concentration declines with chronological age in animals and humans.[108]

Absorption of NMN

NMN is taken up from the gastrointestinal tract into the bloodstream in approximately 2-3 minutes and subsequently delivered to tissues within 10-30 minutes.[102] Following this, NMN is promptly used for the biosynthesis of NAD^+, leading to a notable rise in NAD^+ levels in tissues over the course of 60 minutes. This rapid pharmacokinetic profile has been recently validated through the use of doubly labelled isotopic NMN (C13-D-NMN), which demonstrates its swift absorption and transformation into NAD^+ in peripheral tissues.[102]

The solute carrier family 12 member 8 (Slc12a8) gene encodes a unique NMN transporter found in mammals. The mRNA expression of the Slc12a8 gene increases in response to a decrease in NAD^+, enabling cells to fulfil an urgent and immediate need for NAD^+ biosynthesis. The Slc12a8 NMN transporter is specific and selective for NMN and requires sodium ions for the transport of NMN.[102] The role of the Slc12a8 NMN transporter is particularly important in older adults as opposed to younger individuals. In response to marked reductions in NAD^+ concentrations, the ileum of aged individuals enhances the expression of Slc12a8 in an effort to sustain its NAD^+ levels.[102] When sufficient NMN is provided, this feedback mechanism can operate effectively to preserve NAD^+ levels similar to those found in young ilea. Consequently, augmenting NMN availability or activating the NMN transporter could serve as an effective strategy to mitigate the decline of NAD^+ associated with ageing in the small intestine of older individuals.[102] Whereas nicotinamide riboside is transported into the cell by equilibrative nucleoside transporters (ENTs). Inside the cell, nicotinamide riboside is phosphorylated by nicotinamide riboside kinase (NMRK1 and NMRK2, collectively known as NRK1/2), resulting in the production of NMN. This NMN is then converted into NAD^+ via the activity of nicotinamide mononucleotide adenylyltransferases (NMNATs).[97]

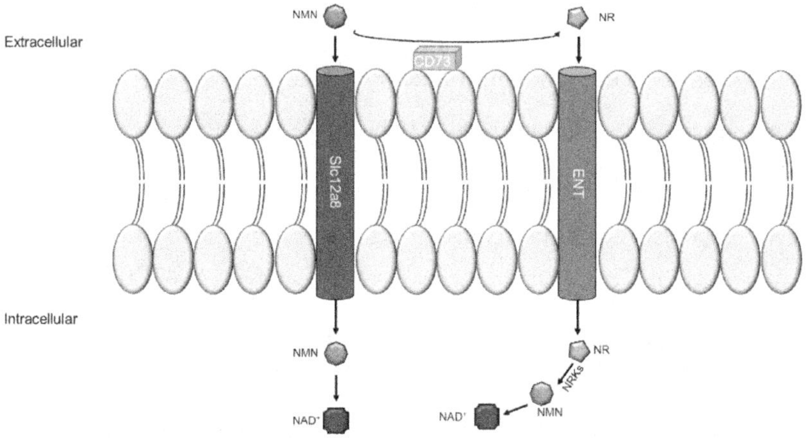

Figure 4. Transportation of NMN and NR into the cell (figure based on references[97,98])

Abbreviations: CD73, cluster of differentiation 73; ENT, equilibrative nucleoside transporters; NAD, nicotinamide adenine dinucleotide; NMN, nicotinamide mononucleotide; NR, nicotinamide riboside; NRKs, nicotinamide riboside kinase; Slc12a8, solute carrier family 12 member 8.

Functions of NMN

In vitro and preclinical research have outlined the various roles of NMN. Below is a non-exhaustive list of the functions of NMN:

- Enhances NAD^+ biosynthesis[42,46,49]
- Increases NAD^+ levels[40-46]
- Increases cellular energy[47]
- Improves mitochondrial bioenergetics[44]
- Energy metabolism[43]
- Increases energy expenditure[46]
- Increased oxygen consumption[46]
- Decreased respiratory quotient[46]

- Improves mitochondrial dynamics[44]
- Improves mitochondrial function[40,49]
- Improve cellular glucose metabolism[40]
- Improves insulin action[46]
- Increases insulin sensitivity[46]
- Improves insulin secretion[46]
- Improves impairments in glucose-stimulated insulin secretion[46]
- Improves cellular lipid metabolism[40]
- Protects the heart from ischaemia/reperfusion injury[45]
- Reduces the infarct area in the heart after ischaemia/reperfusion injury[45]
- Reduces age-related arterial stiffness[50]
- Reduces arterial collagen type I (involved in arterial stiffness)[50]
- Improves endothelial function[50]
- Promotes vascular endothelial formation[42]
- Reduces adipose abdominal fat tissue size[49]
- Cardioprotective[45]
- Reduced age-associated body weight gain[46]
- Improves age-associated increase in adipose tissue inflammation[46]
- Improves eye function[46]
- Increases bone density[46]
- Improves ovary quality[49]
- Reduced meiotic defects and DNA damage in oocytes (ovary cells)[49]
- Stimulates autophagy[45]

- Activates SIRT1[42,50]
- Improves depletion of the NAD^+/SIRT1 pathway[42]
- Anti-inflammatory[41,42,48]
- Decreases inflammatory markers (IL-6, IL-1β and TNF-α)[42]
- Antioxidant[42,43]
- Reduces reactive oxygen species (ROS)[41,43,49]
- Reduces oxidative stress[41,42]
- Reduces vascular oxidative stress[50]
- Neuroprotection[42,43]
- Improves cell viability[41]
- Increases NMN levels[46]
- Potential anti-ageing effects[42]
- Shows potential in memory[42,43] and learning[43]

Human clinical trials of NMN

NMN has numerous important functions in the body. This section explores and presents the various functions of NMN, supported by findings from human clinical trials:

- precursor of NAD^+[47,97,102]
- increases intracellular NAD^+ levels[98,101]
- enhances NAD levels[39,97,108-113]
- enhances muscle insulin signalling[110]
- improves muscle insulin sensitivity[110]
- improves arterial stiffness[114]
- enhances muscle NAD+ turnover[110]
- decreases postprandial hyperinsulinaemia[101]
- decreases total cholesterol[112]
- decreases LDL cholesterol[112]
- decreases apolipoprotein B levels[112]
- decreases diastolic blood pressure[112]
- improves motor function[115]
- improves walking speed[109,115]
- increases walking distance[108,111]
- enhances aerobic capacity[116]
- potential to improve maximal voluntary muscle strength[112]
- shows potential in reducing body weight[112]
- improved sleep quality[109]
- improves longevity[111]
- improves health-related quality of life[108,111]

NMN enhances NAD^+ levels

Nicotinamide mononucleotide enhances NAD^+ levels. A single-centre, single-arm, open-label trial investigated the effect of 125 mg daily on NAD^+ levels in healthy, middle-aged Japanese men.[101] After 8 weeks, NMN administration showed an increase in NAD+ levels in peripheral blood mononuclear cells.[101] Additionally, NMN supplementation was well-tolerated.[101]

A randomised, double-blind, placebo-controlled, parallel trial examined the effects of NMN on blood levels of NAD^+ metabolites, SIRT1 expression, and metabolic health parameters, including cardiovascular disease risk factors. Middle-aged participants took one capsule of either 125 mg NMN or a placebo twice daily for 12 weeks.[114] Nicotinamide levels in the NMN intake group were significantly higher after the intervention compared to the placebo group ($p = 0.037$). Additionally, an intra-group comparison before and after the intervention showed that serum nicotinamide in the NMN group significantly increased after 12 weeks ($p = 0.006$), while in the placebo group it significantly decreased following the intervention ($p = 0.014$). NMN supplementation at 250 mg/day was well tolerated and did not cause adverse events. There were no significant changes in parameters such as haematology, clinical chemistry, and hormones after the 12-week intervention.[114] This study is included in this book due to interest in the effect of NMN supplementation on NAD+ metabolites, specifically nicotinamide.

A randomised, double-blind, placebo-controlled, parallel-group study investigated the safety and efficacy of NMN 250 mg administration in older adults.[115] After 12 weeks, 250 mg of NMN supplementation significantly increased the levels of NMN and NAD^+ in comparison to placebo. NMN at a daily dose of 250 mg for 12 weeks was well tolerated. No notable difference was detected between the NMN and placebo groups concerning haematological and blood chemistry parameters, which include liver enzymes and markers of renal function. Notably, all clinical laboratory values in the NMN group remained within the normal range.[115]

A randomised, double-blind, placebo-controlled, parallel-group comparison trial investigated the effect of 250 mg on levels of NAD^+.[109] There was a significant increase in NAD^+ levels after 12 weeks of NMN. There were no significant changes in blood haematological and biological parameters between the NMN and placebo groups.[109]

A 10-week, randomised, double-blind, placebo-controlled study examined postmenopausal women with prediabetes who were either overweight or obese (body mass index ranging from 25.3 to 39.1 kg/m^2) to assess the impact of NMN 250 mg daily on body composition, insulin sensitivity in skeletal muscle and insulin signalling, the content of muscle NAD^+, as well as the overall gene expression profile.[110] The plasma levels of N-methyl-2-pyridone-5-carboxamide and N-methyl-4-pyridone-5-carboxamide, which are metabolites generated from NMN, showed an increase following 10 weeks of NMN administration, in contrast to the placebo group. Additionally, the basal NAD^+ levels in peripheral blood mononuclear cells (PBMCs) rose after 10 weeks of NMN treatment, whereas no significant changes were observed following placebo treatment.[110]

Eleven healthy participants (20-65 years old, males = 7, females = 4) received 250 mg of NMN once daily in the morning for 12 weeks.

Plasma concentrations of NMN and NAD^+ were measured monthly over 3 months. One month after the participants stopped taking NMN, blood was also collected (month 4). Physiological and laboratory tests were performed within 2 hours after lunch (at 2:00 pm), before and during NMN administration.[39] The concentration of plasma NAD^+ showed a significant increase at 1, 2, and 3 months following the initiation of NMN administration, and then reverted to baseline levels one month after the cessation of NMN intake. The highest NAD^+ concentration was observed after one month of NMN consumption. The concentration of plasma NMN rose significantly as NMN ingestion continued, with the highest concentration observed two months following the initiation of NMN administration. One month after the cessation of NMN intake, the NMN levels reverted to their initial baseline values. It is important to highlight that two participants exhibited significantly elevated NMN concentrations at month 2 and/or month 3, yet did not experience any adverse symptoms.[39] It is important to note that this study includes only 11 participants. A study with a larger sample size could potentially reveal different outcomes regarding NMN and NAD concentrations during and after the study. No adverse symptoms were observed in the participants.[39]

A randomised, multicentre, double-blind, placebo-controlled, parallel-group, dose-dependent clinical trial included 80 middle-aged healthy adults randomly assigned to a 60-day clinical trial with once daily oral dosing of 300 mg NMN, 600 mg NMN, 900 mg NMN, or placebo.[111] Blood NAD levels showed a statistically significant increase from baseline in all three groups treated with NMN at both the 30 and 60-day marks (all $p \leq 0.001$), whereas no significant changes were observed in the placebo group during the same time frames. In comparison to the placebo, blood NAD concentrations were significantly elevated in all three NMN-treated groups at both the 30 and 60-day intervals (all $p < 0.001$). No safety issues were found, based on monitoring adverse events, laboratory and clinical measures, and NMN supplementation was well tolerated.[111]

A multicentre, randomised, double-blind, placebo-controlled, parallel, dose-dependent clinical trial on NMN supplementation on NAD levels.[108] Healthy 40-65 years old individuals ($n = 80$) with a body mass index (BMI) between 18.5-35□kg/m^2 were included in this study. Participants were randomised into four groups receiving daily NMN supplements of 300□mg, 600□mg, and 900□mg, or placebo, for 60 days. Blood NAD concentration, 6-minute walk test, and 36-item short-form survey (SF-36) were measured at baseline and after 60 days. Blood NAD levels increased. The NAD change at both day 30 and day 60 increased dose-dependently ($p<0.001$). The NAD change was dose-dependent with no significant difference between the 600□mg group and the 900□mg NMN group.[108]

A Harvard Medical School study aimed to determine the safety and physiologic effects of NMN (2 x 1,000 mg) daily for 28 days, on a number of physiologic processes including metabolism (body weight, adipose tissue mass in the liver and abdomen, insulin sensitivity), blood pressure, muscle bioenergetics, skeletal muscle performance, physical function, and aerobic capacity in middle-aged and older, overweight or obese adults.[112] NMN resulted in a significant elevation of blood NAD levels from the baseline measurement to days 14 and 28. In contrast, there was no change in blood NAD levels observed within the placebo group. The circulating levels of NAD metabolites, specifically N-methyl-2-

pyridone-5-carboxamide [2-PY], nicotinamide, and 1-methylnicotinamide, were observed to be elevated on days 14 and 28 compared to baseline in the group treated with NMN; however, no changes were noted in the placebo group. There were no serious adverse events. There was no notable difference in the change from baseline regarding liver enzymes (alanine aminotransferase (ALT) and aspartate aminotransferase (AST)), fasting blood glucose, creatinine, uric acid, various blood chemistries, and electrocardiogram metrics (QTc and QRS intervals) among the groups.[112]

A Harvard Medical School randomised, double-blind, placebo-controlled, multiple ascending dose study investigated the effect of NMN on levels of NMN, NAD, and the NAD metabolome.[113] The study participants included overweight or obese individuals (body mass index [BMI] 28-40 kg/m^2), consisting of middle-aged and older men, and postmenopausal women, 55-80 years, all of whom had no significant medical issues. Each participant received tablets containing either 500 mg of NMN or matching placebo tablets, taking either two 500 mg NMN or 2 placebo tablets once daily or twice daily over a period of 14 days. On Days 1 and 14, baseline blood samples were obtained following an overnight fast to measure NMN, NAD, and the NAD metabolome prior to dosing; the study product was administered at time 0; and blood was collected for blood counts and chemistries at 4 hours, as well as for NMN, NAD, and the NAD metabolome at 2, 4, 6, and 24 hours post-administration of the study product. A urine collection over 4 hours was conducted. Blood samples were gathered for pharmacokinetic evaluation of NMN levels and pharmacodynamic assessment (including NAD and the NAD metabolome, which encompasses nicotinamide [NAM], 1-

methyl nicotinamide [1-methyl NAM], N-methyl-2-pyridone-5-carboxamide [2-PY]-NAM, and NR in plasma) prior to dosing (-15 minutes) and at 0, 2, 4, and 24 hours on Day 1; at 0 and 1 hour on Day 8; and prior to dosing (-15 minutes) and at 1, 2, 4, 6, and 24 hours on Day 14. Urine samples were collected for NMN, along with the primary metabolites nicotinamide and 2-PY-NAM, on Days 1 and 14 at 0 and 24 hours. Participants returned on Day 8 for blood counts and chemistries, as well as for the measurement of NMN, NAD, and the NAD metabolome. The treatment of 1,000 mg administered twice daily resulted in a significantly larger increase in NMN levels when compared to the 1,000 mg treatment taken once daily (geometric mean ratios [90% CI] were 1.98 [1.12, 3.48] for C_{max}, which refers to the maximum or peak plasma concentration, and 3.32 [1.14, 9.67] for AUC_{last}, representing the area under the curve from the time of administration until the last quantifiable concentration. A statistically significant difference was observed between the NMN-treated groups and the placebo in terms of blood NMN concentrations on Day 14 ($p = 0.007$ for C_{max} and $p = 0.037$ for AUC_{last}). The once-daily treatment of 1,000 mg was linked to an average increase of 2.7 times and 1.7 times above baseline, while the twice-daily treatment led to increases of 4.5 times and 3.7 times in mean C_{max} and AUC_{last}, respectively, in comparison to the placebo. Participants receiving the 1,000 mg twice-daily treatment exhibited higher NMN C_{max} and AUC_{last} levels than those on the once-daily treatment. NMN treatment was associated with a dose-related increase in blood NAD levels from baseline to Day 14. On Day 1, blood NAD levels showed only a modest increase from baseline to 24 hours in NMN-treated participants. NAD levels were substantially higher on Day 14 than at baseline or Day 1 in participants treated with 1,000 mg once-daily and 1,000 mg twice-daily regimens compared with the placebo group. NAD levels on Day 8 were higher than on Day 1 and were similar to the levels on Day 14 in both NMN dose groups. NAD C_{max} and AUC_{last} on Day 14 were significantly different between the 2 NMN-treated and placebo-treated groups ($p < 0.001$ and $p < 0.001$, respectively). Among the metabolites of NAD present in circulation, 2-PY was found to be the most prevalent. The circulating levels of all four metabolites (2-PY, NAM, 1-methyl NAM, and NR) rose from baseline to 24 hours on Day 1. Furthermore, the concentrations of these metabolites were greater on Days 8 and 14 compared to both Day 1 and baseline in the groups treated with NMN.[113] There were no serious adverse events. Changes from baseline in clinical laboratory analytes in NMN-treated groups did not differ from placebo. There was no clinically significant change from baseline in vital signs or QTc interval in any group.[113] QTc (Corrected QT) refers to the duration required for the heart's ventricles to undergo electrical repolarisation (recharging) following a heartbeat, with adjustments made for heart rate.

NMN improves cardiometabolic health

Nicotinamide mononucleotide has been shown to improve cardiometabolic health via enhanced muscle insulin signalling,[110] improved muscle insulin sensitivity.[110] decreased postprandial hyperinsulinemia,[101] decreased brachial-ankle pulse wave velocity (a marker of vascular stiffness),[114] reduced levels of serum total cholesterol, low-density lipoprotein (LDL) cholesterol, and non-high-density lipoprotein (non-HDL) cholesterol,[112] reduced apolipoprotein B levels,[112] and reduced diastolic blood pressure.[112]

A 10-week, randomised, double-blind, placebo-controlled study examined postmenopausal women with prediabetes who were either overweight or obese (body mass index ranging from 25.3 to 39.1 kg/m^2) to assess the impact of NMN (250 mg daily) supplementation on body composition, insulin sensitivity in skeletal muscle and insulin signalling, the content of muscle NAD^+, as well as the overall gene expression profile.[110] The plasma levels of N-methyl-2-pyridone-5-carboxamide and N-methyl-4-pyridone-5-carboxamide, which are metabolites generated from NMN, showed an increase following 10 weeks of NMN administration, in contrast to the placebo group. Blood NAD levels showed a statistically significant increase from baseline in all three groups treated with NMN at both the 30 and 60-day marks (all $p \leq 0.001$), whereas no significant changes were observed in the placebo group during the same time frames. In comparison to the placebo, blood NAD concentrations were significantly elevated in all three NMN-treated groups at both the 30 and 60-day intervals (all $p < 0.001$). Additionally, the basal NAD^+ levels in peripheral blood mononuclear cells (PBMCs) rose after 10 weeks of NMN treatment, whereas no significant changes were observed following placebo treatment.[110] Furthermore, the concentrations of N-methyl-nicotinamide, methyl-2-pyridone-5-carboxamide, and N-methyl-4-pyridone-5-carboxamide in the quadriceps muscle increased as a result of NMN treatment, but not with placebo treatment, indicating that NMN administration enhances muscle NAD^+ turnover.[110] This study demonstrated that a 10-week treatment of 250 mg of daily NMN supplementation enhances muscle insulin signalling (as evidenced by elevated insulin-stimulated phosphorylated AKT and mammalian target of rapamycin (mTOR)) and improves muscle insulin sensitivity (reflected in the increased insulin-stimulated glucose disposal rate per kg of fat-free mass) among postmenopausal women with prediabetes who are classified as overweight or obese.[110] AKT phosphorylates many proteins involved in polymerisation and stabilisation of the actin cytoskeleton.[117] AKT, commonly referred to as Protein Kinase B (PKB), is a protein kinase that specifically targets serine and threonine residues. It is widely recognised as a pivotal signalling hub that governs numerous cellular processes, such as proliferation, survival, apoptosis, and metabolism.[117] The enhancement in muscle insulin sensitivity holds significant clinical importance.[110] No adverse events were reported, and no abnormalities in standard blood tests were detected in either group.[110]

A single-centre, single-arm, open-label trial investigated the effect of 125 mg daily on postprandial hyperinsulinaemia, a risk factor for coronary artery disease, in healthy, middle-aged Japanese men.[101] After 8 weeks, in participants with insulin over-secretion after oral glucose loading, NMN moderately decreased postprandial hyperinsulinemia.[101] Additionally, NMN supplementation was well-tolerated.[101]

A randomised, double-blind, placebo-controlled, parallel trial examined the effects of NMN on blood levels of NAD+ metabolites, SIRT1 expression, and metabolic health parameters, including cardiovascular disease risk factors. Middle-aged participants took one capsule of either 125 mg NMN or a placebo twice daily for 12 weeks.[114] In individuals with above-average body mass index (BMI) or blood glucose levels, brachial-ankle pulse wave velocity (a marker of arterial stiffness) in the NMN intake group was significantly lower after the test period compared to the placebo group. These findings suggest that NMN supplementation might enhance vascular health in middle-aged adults, especially those with high BMI or blood glucose levels. Furthermore, the results imply that NMN supplementation could reduce vascular stiffness and decrease the risk of cardiovascular disease events. NMN supplementation at 250 mg/day was well tolerated and did not cause adverse events. There were no significant changes in parameters such as haematology, clinical chemistry, and hormones after the 12-week intervention.[114]

A study aimed to determine the safety and physiologic effects of NMN (2 x 1,000 mg) daily for 28 days, on a number of physiologic processes including metabolism (body weight, adipose tissue mass in the liver and abdomen, insulin sensitivity), blood pressure, muscle bioenergetics, skeletal muscle performance, physical function, and aerobic capacity in middle-aged and older, overweight or obese adults.[112] The levels of serum total cholesterol, low-density lipoprotein (LDL) cholesterol, and non-high-density lipoprotein (non-HDL) cholesterol exhibited a reduction from baseline in the NMN group; the differences between groups regarding the change from baseline in total cholesterol (-0.7 [-1.15, -0.24] mmol/L, P = 0.004), LDL (-0.48 [-0.82, -0.14] mmol/L, P = 0.007), and non-HDL (-0.64 [-1.02, -0.25] mmol/L, P = 0.002) were statistically significant. Additionally, apolipoprotein B levels decreased in the NMN group while remaining unchanged in the placebo group. Diastolic blood pressure exhibited a reduction from baseline in the NMN group, whereas no change was observed in the placebo group;

furthermore, the reduction in diastolic blood pressure from baseline was significantly more pronounced in the NMN group compared to the placebo group (difference -7.01 [-13.44, -0.59] mmHg, P = 0.034). There were no serious adverse events. There was no notable difference in the change from baseline regarding liver enzymes (alanine aminotransferase (ALT) and aspartate aminotransferase (AST)), fasting blood glucose, creatinine, uric acid, various blood chemistries, and electrocardiogram metrics (QTc and QRS intervals) among the groups.[112]

NMN improves motor function, walking speed, and walking distance

Nicotinamide mononucleotide has been shown to improve motor function, walking speed, and walking distance. A randomised, double-blind, placebo-controlled, parallel-group study investigated the safety and efficacy of NMN administration in older adults.[115] After 6 weeks, there was a significant improvement in both gait speed and the left grip assessment. The gait speed evaluation quantifies the duration required for an individual to walk a predetermined short distance, in this case, 10 metres. It serves as a straightforward, cost-effective, and dependable measure of an individual's overall physical function and health condition. The objective of the handgrip strength assessment is to evaluate the peak isometric strength of the muscles in the hand and forearm. Furthermore, a significant difference was noted in the outcomes of the 30-second chair-stand assessment between the NMN and placebo groups following the 6 week period. The 30-second chair-stand test measures the number of times a participant can stand up and sit down from the standard chair without armrests in 30 seconds. NMN at a daily dose of 250 mg for 12 weeks was well tolerated. No notable difference was detected between the NMN and placebo groups concerning haematological and blood chemistry parameters, which include liver enzymes and markers of renal function. Notably, all clinical laboratory values in the NMN group remained within the normal range.[115]

A randomised, double-blind, placebo-controlled, parallel-group comparison trial investigated the effect of 250 mg on motor function.[109] After 12 weeks, the NMN group had a significantly faster 4 metre walking time than the placebo group. A significant inverse relationship was observed with the 4-metre walking test duration and the variations in blood NAD^+, N1-methyl-2-pyridone-5-carboxamide (2-PY), and N1-methyl-4-pyridone-3-carboxamide (4-PY) after 12 weeks of 250 mg of NMN. There were no significant changes in blood haematological and biological parameters between the NMN and placebo groups.[109]

A randomised, multicentre, double-blind, placebo-controlled, parallel-group, dose-dependent clinical trial included 80 middle-aged healthy adults randomly assigned to a 60-day clinical trial with once daily oral dosing of 300 mg NMN, 600 mg NMN, 900 mg NMN, or placebo.[111] Walking distance increase during the six-minute walking test was statistically significantly higher in the 300 mg, 600 mg, and 900 mg groups compared to placebo at both days 30 and 60 (all $p < 0.01$), with the longest walking distances measured in the 600 mg and 900 mg groups. Participants in the 600 mg NMN-treated group had a statistically longer walking distance compared to the 300 mg NMN-treated group at days 30 and 60 (both $p < 0.01$). There was no statistical difference in the walking distance between the 900 mg and 600 mg NMN-treated group (both p >

0.05). No safety issues, based on monitoring adverse events, laboratory and clinical measures, were found, and NMN supplementation was well tolerated.[111]

A multicentre, randomised, double-blind, placebo-controlled, parallel, dose-dependent clinical trial on NMN supplementation on 6-minute walking test.[108] Healthy 40-65 years old individuals (n = 80) with a body mass index (BMI) between 18.5-35□kg/m2 were included in this study. Participants were randomised into four groups receiving daily NMN supplements of 300□mg, 600□mg, and 900□mg, or placebo, for 60 days. Blood NAD concentration, 6-minute walk test, and 36-item short-form survey (SF-36) were measured at baseline and after 60 days. A greater change in NAD levels was significantly linked to enhanced improvement in the 6-minute walk test at both day 30 and day 60. Specifically, for every 1 nmol/L rise in blood NAD concentration at day 30, there was a corresponding increase of 1.37 m in the 6-minute walk test. Furthermore, each unit increase in NAD levels on day 60 correlated with an additional 2.42 m in the 6-minute walk test. The 6-minute walk test serves as a tool for evaluating the advancement of functional exercise capacity in clinical intervention research. An elevation in blood NAD concentration correlated with an enhancement in the 6-minute walking distance, indicating improved physical performance.[108]

NMN enhances aerobic capacity

Nicotinamide mononucleotide has been shown to enhance aerobic capacity. Consistent physical activity enhances aerobic capacity, cardiovascular health, metabolic function, and overall physical performance; however, numerous enhancements may be associated with NAD^+/sirtuins.[116] Engaging in exercise training elevates the expression of nicotinamide phosphoribosyltransferase (NAMPT), which is the rate-limiting enzyme in the NAD^+ salvage pathway, alongside increasing NAD^+ levels and sirtuin activity. Endurance athletes exhibit elevated NAMPT expression in their skeletal muscle.[116] A randomised, double-blind, placebo-controlled, four-arm clinical trial was conducted to investigate the effects of NMN on aerobic capacity in amateur runners.[116] The participants were randomised into four groups: the low dosage group (NMN 150 mg twice daily), the medium dosage group (NMN 300 mg twice daily), the high dosage group (NMN 600 mg twice daily), and the control group (placebo). Each group consisted of ten male participants and two female participants. After 6 weeks, the oxygen uptake (VO_2), the percentages of maximum oxygen uptake (VO_2max), as well as the power at the first and second ventilatory thresholds, exhibited a more significant increase in the medium (NMN 300 mg twice daily) and high dosage (NMN 600 mg twice daily) groups in comparison to the control group.[116] The findings suggest that NMN supplementation significantly enhanced the ventilatory threshold beyond what was achieved through exercise alone.[116] The combination of exercise training and NMN supplementation could represent an innovative and effective approach to enhance the endurance performance of athletes.[116]

NMN shows potential in improving maximal voluntary muscle strength

Nicotinamide mononucleotide has been shown to improve maximal voluntary muscle strength. A study aimed to determine the safety and physiologic effects of NMN (2 x 1,000 mg) daily for 28 days, on a number of physiologic processes including metabolism (body weight, adipose tissue mass in the liver and abdomen, insulin sensitivity), blood pressure, muscle bioenergetics, skeletal muscle performance, physical function, and aerobic capacity in middle-aged and older, overweight or obese adults.[112] The maximal voluntary muscle strength, measured as the 1-repetition maximum in both leg press and chest press exercises, along with muscle fatigability, assessed through repetitions to failure in these same exercises, as well as stair-climbing power, demonstrated numerically larger increases in the NMN group compared to the placebo group; however, the differences between the groups did not reach statistical significance. There were no serious adverse events. There was no notable difference in the change from baseline regarding liver enzymes (alanine aminotransferase (ALT) and aspartate aminotransferase (AST)), fasting blood glucose, creatinine, uric acid, various blood chemistries, and electrocardiogram metrics (QTc and QRS intervals) among the groups.[112]

NMN shows potential in reducing body weight

Nicotinamide mononucleotide has the potential to be utilised in programs for reducing body weight. A study aimed to determine the safety and physiologic effects of NMN (2 x 1,000 mg) daily for 28 days, on a number of physiologic processes including metabolism (body weight, adipose tissue mass in the liver and abdomen, insulin sensitivity), blood pressure, muscle bioenergetics, skeletal muscle performance, physical function, and aerobic capacity in middle-aged and older, overweight or obese adults.[112] Participants in the NMN group experienced a reduction in body weight, whereas those in the placebo group saw an increase; the difference in body weight change between the two groups was statistically significant (difference = -1.9 kg, 95% CI -3.3, -0.5, P = 0.008). There were no serious adverse events. There was no notable difference in the change from baseline regarding liver enzymes (alanine aminotransferase (ALT) and aspartate aminotransferase (AST)), fasting blood glucose, creatinine, uric acid, various blood chemistries, and electrocardiogram metrics (QTc and QRS intervals) among the groups.[112]

NMN improves sleep quality

Nicotinamide mononucleotide has been shown to improve sleep quality. A randomised, double-blind, placebo-controlled, parallel-group comparison trial investigated the effect of 250 mg on sleep quality.[109] The Pittsburgh Sleep Quality Index (PSQI) assesses sleep quality and disturbances over a one-month time interval. The PSQI scores pertaining to "Daytime dysfunction" and "Global PSQI" were markedly lower in the NMN group compared to the placebo group at the 12-week point. At the 4-week point, those participants in the NMN group had a significantly lower score for "Global PSQI" compared to the placebo group.[109] There were no significant changes in blood haematological and biological parameters between the NMN and placebo groups.[109]

NMN, Ageing, and Longevity

Nicotinamide mononucleotide has the potential to enhance healthy ageing and longevity. The levels of NAD^+ decline in numerous tissues as one ages,[101,102] including skeletal muscle, liver, adipose tissue, brain, pancreas, spleen, heart, kidney, and lung, which contributes to the emergence of various pathophysiological conditions associated with ageing.[102] This decline is attributed, at least in part, to two molecular processes: the reduction in NAD^+ biosynthesis linked to nicotinamide phosphoribosyltransferase (NAMPT), which is the rate-limiting enzyme for NAD^+ production in mammals, and the increase in NAD^+ consumption due to NAD^+-utilising enzymes, such as poly-ADP-ribose polymerases (PARPS) and CD38.[102]

NMN serves as a biosynthetic precursor to NAD^+ that is recognised for its ability to enhance cellular NAD^+ synthesis and counteract age-related disorders linked to a reduction in tissue NAD^+ concentrations.[102]

A randomised, multicentre, double-blind, placebo-controlled, parallel-group, dose-dependent clinical trial included 80 middle-aged healthy adults randomly assigned to a 60-day clinical trial with once daily oral dosing of 300 mg NMN, 600 mg NMN, 900 mg NMN, or placebo.[111] The blood biological age increased significantly in the placebo group and stayed unchanged in all NMN-treated groups at day 60, which resulted in a significant difference between the treated groups and placebo (all $p < 0.05$). No safety issues, based on monitoring adverse events, laboratory and clinical measures, were found, and NMN supplementation was well tolerated.[111]

NMN improves quality of life

Nicotinamide mononucleotide has been shown to improve health-related quality of life. A randomised, multicentre, double-blind, placebo-controlled, parallel-group, dose-dependent clinical trial included 80 middle-aged healthy adults randomly assigned to a 60-day clinical trial with once daily oral dosing of 300 mg NMN, 600 mg NMN, 900 mg NMN, or placebo.[111] The SF-36 measures eight scales: physical functioning, role physical, bodily pain, general health, vitality, social functioning, role emotional, and mental health.[118] In comparison to the placebo, all three groups treated with NMN exhibited significantly improved SF-36 scores at day 60 ($p < 0.01$), as well as the 600 mg and 900 mg groups at day 30 ($p < 0.05$ and $p < 0.001$, respectively). No safety issues, based on monitoring adverse events, laboratory and clinical measures, were found, and NMN supplementation was well tolerated.[111]

A multicentre, randomised, double-blind, placebo-controlled, parallel, dose-dependent clinical trial on NMN supplementation on health-related quality of life.[108] Healthy 40-65 years old individuals ($n = 80$) with a body mass index (BMI) between 18.5-35□kg/m^2 were included in this study. Participants were randomised into four groups receiving daily NMN supplements of 300 mg, 600 mg, and 900 mg, or placebo, for 60 days. Blood NAD concentration, 6-minute walk test, and 36-item short-form survey (SF-36) were measured at baseline and after 60 days. The SF-36 score serves as a validated instrument for evaluating health-related quality of life. It encompasses eight distinct domains, each with its own scoring: physical functioning, role physical, bodily pain, general health, vitality, social functioning, role emotional, and mental health. A greater change in NAD was significantly correlated with enhanced improvement in the SF-36 score change at both day 30 and day 60.[108]

Daily dosage ranges for NMN supplementation

Human studies involving NMN have documented a range of daily dosages, including: 100 mg,[119] 125 mg,[101] 250 mg,[39,101,109,110,114,115,119] 300 mg,[108,111,116] 500 mg,[119] 600 mg,[108,111,116] 900 mg,[108,111] 1,000 mg,[112,113] 1,200 mg,[116] 1,250 mg,[120] and 2,000 mg.[112,113]

Safety

Various studies have shown that NMN is well-tolerated,[111-114,119,120] and no safety concerns related to NMN supplementation have been identified,[111,114,119] based on monitoring adverse events, laboratory results, and clinical measures.[111,112,120]

PART 3. NUTRIENT AND HERBAL COMBINATIONS WITH NMN

Potential nutrient combinations with NMN

NMN can be used as a standalone active ingredient or in conjunction with other nutrients. If you're considering taking NMN alongside other products, it's important to reflect on the results you aim to achieve and the underlying mechanisms of action. Some potential benefits include enhanced energy levels, improved immune system function, better cardiovascular health, increased aerobic capacity, and greater longevity.

When creating and formulating products that incorporate NMN along with other nutrients, keep in mind the mechanisms of action and the synergy between the proposed vitamins, minerals, or other nutrients. Utilise your knowledge of nutritional biochemistry, anatomy, physiology, and pathophysiology to guide you in developing a product that meets your desired outcomes.

Vitamins are a group of organic compounds that are essential for normal physiological functioning.[8] Vitamins cannot be synthesised by humans and therefore must be obtained from the diet.[8,121] Vitamins and minerals may be chosen and utilised for their antidepressant,[2] anti-inflammatory,[3-7] antioxidant,[8-10] anti-anxiety (anxiolytic),[2] bone health,[11,12] bone mass,[122] bone mineral density,[122] brain signalling,[13] calcium homeostasis,[123] carbohydrate metabolism,[124,125] cell function,[14,15] coagulation,[121,126-128] collagen synthesis,[121,124] cognitive function,[129] connective tissue,[130,131] differentiation,[132,133] DNA metabolism,[8,16] DNA synthesis,[14,15,124,134] endothelial cell function,[124] energy metabolism.[17,18] enzymatic reactions,[121] fat metabolism,[124] gene expression,[16] gene expression,[133] glucose metabolism,[19,20] glycaemic control,[135] haemoglobin formation,[14] heart rhythm,[136,137] homocysteine metabolism,[8,9] immune system health,[21] insulin secretion,[16] Krebs cycle activity,[17] lipid peroxidation reduction,[138] liver health,[138] methylation processes,[9,14,124,139,140] mitochondrial health,[136] muscle function,[136,141] myelination,[142] nerve function,[136,141,143] nerve conduction and excitability,[144] neuromuscular activity,[145] neurotransmitter metabolism,[146] neurotransmitter synthesis,[121,147] oxidation-reduction reactions,[9,10] protein metabolism,[124,148] red blood cell formation,[15] signal transduction,[142,149] thyroid hormone regulation,[147] thyroid hormone production,[150-154] trans-sulphuration processes,[9,146] and vasodilator[155] functions. This section provides a summary of various vitamins, minerals, and other nutrients that could potentially be taken alongside NMN or be combined in formulations with NMN.

Vitamin B1

Vitamin B1 (Thiamine) is a water-soluble vitamin. Vitamin B1 is involved in the synthesis of nucleic acids,[8] fatty acids,[8] steroids,[8] and contributes to the structure and function of cellular membranes, including neurons and neuroglia,[8] and is involved with cell membrane dynamics,[18] and cell signalling.[18]

Vitamin B1 is involved in energy metabolism.[17,18] It is involved in carbohydrate,[124,125] protein, and fat metabolism,[124] and the metabolism of glucose.[156]

Vitamin B1 is involved in the synthesis of the aromatic amino acid precursors to a range of neurotransmitters,[8] metabolism of the neurotransmitter acetylcholine,[8] and has a neuro-modulatory role in the acetylcholine neurotransmitter system.[8] It is involved in nerve structure and function,[157] plays an important role in nerve conduction and excitability,[144] use of glucose by nervous tissue,[147]

Vitamin B2

Vitamin B2 (Riboflavin) is a water-soluble vitamin. Vitamin B2 is involved in cellular development,[15] essential for normal cell function,[14,15] and oxidation-reduction reactions.[9,10] It is a component of two important coenzymes: flavin mononucleotide (FMN) and flavin adenine dinucleotide (FAD).[15] FMN and FAD act as electron carriers.[9] Vitamin B2 is involved in the normal functioning of glutathione reductase,[158] as a cofactor for methylenetetrahydrofolate reductase (MTHFR).[9] It is involved in the conversion of methylenetetrahydrofolate (MTHF) to methyltetrahydrofolate (5-MTHF) by the enzyme MTHFR.[8,9,124] It is also involved in the metabolism of fats[15] and fatty acid synthesis.[124] It is essential for normal growth[14] for the synthesis of all haem proteins, including haemoglobin, nitric oxide synthases, and P450 enzymes.[8] and the synthesis of proteins involved in electron transfer.[8]

As an antioxidant,[8-10] Flavin adenine dinucleotide (FAD) transports hydrogen from NADPH to oxidised glutathione to convert it into the reduced (antioxidant) form[10] to be utilised. It is involved in the glutathione redox cycle[10] and increases endogenous antioxidant status as essential cofactors in the glutathione redox cycle. [8] Vitamin B2 is involved in oxidation-reduction reactions.[9,10]

Vitamin B2 is involved in energy metabolism,[9,14,15] metabolism of carbohydrates, amino acids, and lipids,[14] catabolism of fuel molecules (e.g., ß-oxidation of fatty acids, Krebs cycle),[124] as an essential co-enzyme in mitochondrial aerobic respiration and cellular energy production via direct role in the Krebs cycle, the electron transport chain, and the resultant formation of adenosine triphosphate (ATP), [8] the molecule the body uses for energy. It is involved in the synthesis of proteins involved in electron transfer.[8]

Vitamin B2 is required for the normal functioning of the cardiovascular system. [158] It is involved in the synthesis of proteins involved in oxygen transport and storage,[8] synthesis of all haem proteins, including haemoglobin and nitric oxide synthases,[8] and in the metabolism of homocysteine.[9]

Vitamin B3

Vitamin B3 (Nicotinamide, Nicotinic acid)is generally not combined with NMN. Nicotinamide, a neutral uncharged molecule, rapidly permeates and diffuses across plasma and mitochondrial membranes.[95] It is noted that both nicotinamide and nicotinic acid exhibit synergistic effects in increasing NAD^+ levels within cells.[95]

Vitamin B3 is involved in energy metabolism[8,16,124] and in enzymes involved in oxidation of fuel substrates[124] It is an essential co-enzyme in mitochondrial aerobic respiration and cellular energy production via direct role in the Krebs cycle, the electron transport chain, and the resultant formation of adenosine triphosphate (ATP).[8]

Vitamin B3 is involved in the modulation of inflammation[8,16,138] and modulation of inflammatory cascades.[8] As an antioxidant, it works in antioxidant protection,[8] reduces oxidative stress,[16,138] and reduces lipid peroxidation. [138] Vitamin B3 is a vasodilator.[155] It reduces triglyceride levels,[159] modulates insulin secretion,[16] reduces lipid peroxidation,[138] and is involved in anti-atherogenic lipolysis in adipose tissue.[8]

Vitamin B5

Vitamin B5 (Pantothenic acid) is a water-soluble vitamin. Vitamin B5 is involved in the synthesis of fatty acids,[8,124] membrane phospholipids,[8,124] amino acids,[8,124] porphyrin and corrin rings, [124] and steroid hormones.[8,124] It is needed for acetylation and acylation of proteins[124] and for oxidative metabolism.[8] Vitamin B5 is involved in the synthesis of cholesterol[8] and fatty acids.[8]

Vitamin B5 is involved in the generation of cellular energy and energy metabolism.[8] It is essential co-enzyme in mitochondrial aerobic respiration and cellular energy production via direct role in the Krebs cycle, the electron transport chain, and the resultant formation of adenosine triphosphate (ATP).[8] Vitamin B5 is involved in the synthesis of neurotransmitters.[8,124]

Vitamin B6

Vitamin B6 (Pyridoxine) is a water-soluble vitamin with 3 primary forms: pyridoxine, pyridoxal, and pyridoxamine.[121] Vitamin B6 participates in more than 100 enzymatic reactions.[121] It is an essential cofactor in the functioning of over 140 separate enzymes required for the synthesis, degradation, and interconversion of amino acids.[8] The active form, Pyridoxyl-5-phosphate (PLP), is a cofactor in more than 160 different catalytic functions[146] Vitamin B6 is essential for protein metabolism[14,121] and is a coenzyme in the metabolism of amino acids, glycogen, and sphingoid bases.[124] It is involved in decarboxylation and transamination processes,[155] metabolism of one-carbon units,[14,146] metabolism of carbohydrates and lipids,[14] and is involved in gluconeogenesis,[14] trans-sulphuration processes,[9,146] and in the formation of haemoglobin.[14] It is involved in the conversion of tryptophan to niacin.[14,121,160]

Vitamin B6 is involved in the formation of haemoglobin,[14] metabolism of homocysteine via trans-sulphuration,[9] and trans-sulphuration processes.[9,146]

Vitamin B6 plays a role in nervous system health. It is involved in neurological development,[14] synthesis of neurotransmitters,[121,147] and plays an important role in nerve conduction and excitability.[144] PLP plays an important role in the metabolism of neurotransmitters, such as dopamine, serotonin, glutamate, and gamma-aminobutyric acid (GABA).[146] Vitamin B6 improves dream recall.[161] Vitamin B6 supports a Th1 cytokine-mediated immune response and modulates immune cell function.[162]

Folate

Folate is an essential water-soluble vitamin.[163] The supplemental forms include folic acid and folinic acid,[164] and the active forms of methylfolate 5-MTHF (calcium-l-methylfolate[165] and (6S)-5-methyltetrahydrofolic acid glucosamine[165]).

Folate is involved in one-carbon metabolism,[139,140,163,166-169] metabolism of amino acids,[14,15] methylation processes,[9,14,124,139,140] genomic and non-genomic methylation reactions,[8] synthesis of DNA,[15,163,166,167,170] methylation of DNA,[14,121,163] DNA repair,[167] and reduces DNA damage.[124] It is involved in the synthesis of RNA,[15,166] purines and pyrimidines,[14,140] proteins[166] re-methylation of homocysteine to methionine,[9,139,140] methionine regeneration,[121,124] involved with the synthesis of S-adenosylmethionine (SAMe),[124] and integrity of membrane phospholipids.[8] Folate can influence telomere length and function.[167] The effects of folate on telomeres could be due to its role in DNA synthesis and repair, and one-carbon metabolism within the cell.[167]

Folate is necessary for embryogenesis[121] and foetal development.[8,124] folate is necessary for the production of red blood cells (erythropoiesis),[121] and improved endothelial cell function.[124] Folate is involved in amine and catecholamine neurotransmitter synthesis,[8] and the synthesis and regeneration of tetrahydrobiopterin, an essential cofactor for the enzymes that convert amino acids to both monoamine neurotransmitters (serotonin, melatonin, dopamine, adrenaline, noradrenaline).[8] It is involved in myelination.[8]

Vitamin B12

Vitamin B12 is a water-soluble vitamin. The forms of Vitamin B12 include cyanocobalamin and the active forms of methylcobalamin, 5-deoxyadenosylcobalamin, and hydroxocobalamin. Vitamin B12 is involved in DNA synthesis,[14,15,124,134] regulation of DNA,[14,134] synthesis of RNA,[15] normal synthesis of purines and pyrimidines,[14] protein synthesis,[15] fatty acid synthesis,[14] methylation,[9] blood cell formation,[171] cell metabolism,[14] and for the integrity of membrane phospholipids.[8] It is a cofactor for methionine synthase.[15]

Vitamin B12 is involved in energy metabolism.[14] Vitamin B12 is necessary for red blood cell formation,[15] essential for normal blood function,[124] and is involved in the metabolism of homocysteine.[8,9,171]

Vitamin B12 is essential for the normal functioning of the nervous system[171] and is essential for normal neurological function.[15,124] It is involved in the synthesis of neurotransmitters,[147] genomic and non-genomic methylation reactions in brain tissue,[8] myelin synthesis[171] and myelination.[8] It has an important role in nerve conduction and excitability[144] Vitamin B12 has been associated with improvement of cognitive functions, especially in the elderly.[147]

Biotin

Biotin is a water-soluble vitamin.[172] Biotin plays important roles in a variety of critical metabolic reactions in the cell and is essential for normal human health, growth, and development.[173]

Biotin is essential for cellular metabolism, proliferation, and survival.[174] It plays a role as a coenzyme for carboxylase enzymes.[15,172,174,175] Biotin is involved in carboxylation reactions[155] and regulation of gene expression,[15,172,174,176] where expression of over 2,000 human genes appears to be affected by biotin status.[174] Biotin catalyses fundamental steps in the metabolism of glucose, amino acids and fatty acids,[15,172,174,175] metabolism of branched-chain amino acids,[177] involved in gluconeogenesis,[175] is necessary for fatty acid synthesis,[172,175,177] regulates mitochondrial fatty acid transport[172] is involved in cell signalling,[15] involved with direct interaction with histones and other molecules[172] and histone modification,[15] and plays an essential role in acute oxygen (O_2) sensing[172] and epidermal differentiation.[155]

Biotin is involved in cellular energy metabolism (i.e., ATP production),[174] mitochondrial function,[176] plays a key role in glucose metabolism and haemostasis,[8] gluconeogenesis[8,177] regulates tricarboxylic acid (TCA) intermediates (oxalacetate, succinyl-CoA and acetyl-CoA),[172] and in the regulation of hepatic glucose uptake[8]

Vitamin C

Vitamin C is a water-soluble vitamin. Vitamin C is required for normal physiological functions.[178] It acts as a cofactor in hydroxylation reactions, which are required for collagen synthesis[121,124] and is involved in the synthesis and metabolism of collagen,[14] catecholamines,[14] carnitine,[14,124] and the metabolism of tyrosine,[14,124,178] along with the hydroxylation of glycine, proline, lysine,[178] carnitine,[14,178] and catecholamines.[178]

Vitamin C has anti-inflammatory properties.[179] It is an antioxidant[15,121,124,178,180,181] with free radical scavenging effects.[180] It is involved in the maintenance of glutathione in the reduced form.[124] Vitamin C stimulates the synthesis and activation of antioxidant enzymes, such as superoxide dismutase, glutathione peroxidase, and catalase.[180] It interacts with other antioxidants, including tocopherol, glutathione and thioredoxin,[180] and aids in the regeneration of tocopherol (vitamin E).[124,182] It potentially protects lipids[124] and low-density lipoproteins against oxidative damage.[15,124]

Vitamin C facilitates the conversion of cholesterol into bile acids.[178] Vitamin C plays an essential role in the intestinal absorption of iron[15,121,124,178] due to its chelating and reducing effect, assisting the mobilisation of iron, and intestinal iron absorption[15]

Vitamin C is involved in the synthesis and metabolism of collagen.[14] It acts as a cofactor in hydroxylation reactions of lysine and proline, which are required for collagen synthesis.[15,121,124] Vitamin C increases wound healing.[121]

Vitamin C modulates immune cell function and supports Th1 cytokine-mediated immune responses,[162] enhances neutrophil chemotaxis and T-lymphocyte proliferation in response to infection,[179] and increases cytokine production and synthesis of immunoglobulins.[179]

Vitamin D3

Vitamin D is a fat-soluble vitamin.[15] Vitamin D is involved in differentiation,[132,133] gene expression,[133] regulation of gene transcription,[133] growth and differentiation of keratinocytes through binding to the nuclear vitamin D receptor.[15] It is involved in overall metabolic function[183] and plays an important role in maintaining adequate serum levels of calcium and phosphorus.[15] Vitamin D and its metabolites are steroid hormones and hormone precursors[132]

Vitamin D has anti-inflammatory properties[15] and has a clinical application in chronic inflammatory diseases.[124,133]

Vitamin D has effects on myocardial contractility,[184] and improves vascular compliance.[135] It improves glycaemic control[135] by the stimulation of insulin production[184] and by improving insulin sensitivity[135,183]

Vitamin D is essential for neuromuscular activity.[145] It has a neuroprotective role[133] and induces remyelination.[133] Vitamin D has antidepressant[2] and anxiolytic effects.[2] Research has shown that vitamin D supplementation can lead to an increase in serum serotonin levels in individuals with depression.[2] A correlation has been observed between lower serum vitamin D levels and symptoms of depression and anxiety.[2]

Vitamin D improves bone health,[124] regulates bone turnover,[121,133] and is involved in bone metabolism.[121,132,133,185] It enhances mineralisation of bone,[135] increases bone mineral density[121,184] and bone mineral content,[124] and improves peak bone mass.[184] Vitamin D is involved in optimal muscle function,[133] improves and maintains muscle strength,[124,145] and is essential for neuromuscular activity.[145]

Vitamin D maintains the immune system.[124,133] It has an immunoregulatory role,[15,133] plays an essential role in both cell-mediated and humoral antibody response,[162] and is involved in the modulation of activated T and B lymphocyte function.[184] It regulates the immune system response,[179] increases the oxidative burst potential of macrophages,[179] stimulates natural killer cells,[133] and stimulates the expression of potent anti-microbial peptides.

Vitamin E Tocotrienols

Vitamin E has eight different isoforms that belong to two categories, tocopherols and tocotrienols. There are four saturated analogues of vitamin E, being the tocopherols alpha (α), beta (β), gamma (γ) and delta (δ) and four unsaturated analogues alpha (α), beta (β), gamma (γ) and delta (δ), which are the tocotrienols.[3,4,186-189] I like tocotrienols as they are more readily transferred and incorporated into cell membranes than tocopherols.[3,189] The cellular uptake of tocotrienols is up to 70 times higher than that of tocopherols[3] Vitamin E increases cell viability[182] and has anti-inflammatory effects.[3-7]

Vitamin E is an antioxidant.[3,5-7,14,121,124,181,186,187,190-193] The antioxidant activities of tocotrienols are mediated through induction of various antioxidant enzymes, such as superoxide dismutase and glutathione peroxidase.[3] It is a free radical scavenger.[14,121,181] Vitamin E reduces oxidative protein damage,[187,193] protects cell membranes from oxidative damage,[14] reduces oxidative damage to lipid membranes and low-density lipoprotein (LDL) cholesterol,[121,124] and reduces lipid peroxidation.[182,194] Tocotrienols have been shown to have 40-60 times higher antioxidant activity against induced lipid peroxidation than tocopherols.[3] Tocotrienols are neuroprotective[7,186-188,191,195] and have nervous system membrane protection properties.[147]

Vitamin E tocotrienols have cholesterol-lowering properties.[4,6,196] The mechanism of action of the cholesterol-lowering properties of tocotrienols is via inhibition of HMG-CoA reductase (3-hydroxy-3-methylglutaryl coenzyme A reductase), an enzyme that is rate-limiting in the pathway to cholesterol biosynthesis.[3,187,193,197] Vitamin E also has hypoglycaemic effects (lowering blood glucose levels)[5] and reducing platelet adhesion properties.[121]

Vitamin K2

Vitamin K is a fat-soluble vitamin.[128,198,199] Vitamin K2 is involved in calcium transport,[127] calcium homeostasis,[123] synthesis of matrix Gla protein,[127,200-202] cofactor for carboxylation of glutamate to gamma carboxyglutamic acid (Gla),[127] activation of matrix Gla protein,[198,202] decreases desphospho-uncarboxylated MGP (dp-ucMGP),[203,204] production of osteocalcin,[128,201] activates osteocalcin,[13] carboxylation of osteocalcin,[12,128,205-207] and acts as a transcriptional regulator.[13]

Vitamin K2 has anti-inflammatory[126] and antioxidant properties.[13] It regulates adipokine levels[126] and is involved in energy metabolism.[13] Vitamin K2 has immunomodulatory properties[13]

Vitamin K2 improves cardiometabolic health.[126] It is involved in coagulation[121,126-128] and is essential for the production of prothrombin and coagulation factors.[121,201] It is involved in the gamma-carboxylation of coagulation proteins.[155] It has lipid-lowering effects.[126] Vitamin K2 prevents calcium deposition in the lining of blood vessel walls,[127,128,202] reducing arterial stiffening,[128] and prevents soft tissue calcification.[127]

Vitamin K2 is involved in brain signalling,[13] synthesis of sphingolipids in the brain,[127] and regulation of sphingolipid metabolism.[13] It activates growth arrest-specific protein 6 (Gas6), which is widely present in the nervous system and regulates neuroinflammation.[13]

Vitamin K2 is involved in bone health.[11,12] It is necessary for normal bone metabolism.[121] It improves bone density and bone quality,[127] bone mineralisation,[128] regulation of osteocalcin (synthesised in bone),[127,200] and converts undercarboxylated osteocalcin to carboxylated osteocalcin.[208] It is involved in the gamma-carboxylation of bone proteins,[155] and synthesis of matrix GLa protein (synthesised in cartilage and in blood vessel walls).[127,200,201] It binds and activates the steroid and xenobiotic receptor in order to mediate transcription in bone tissue[155] Vitamin K2 prevents soft tissue calcification.[127]

Chromium

Chromium (Cr) is a micromineral. Chromium is involved in the metabolism of carbohydrates,[148,209] glucose,[19,20] lipids,[20,148,209] protein,[148] and insulin.[20] Chromium also increases the efficiency of insulin.[148]

Research on chromium has found reduced insulin requirements for people with hyperglycaemia.[210] Additionally, chromium decreases cholesterol levels,[211] decreases very low-density lipoprotein-cholesterol (VLDL)[211] and serum triglycerides,[211] and has been found to improve glucose tolerance in women with polycystic ovary syndrome (PCOS).[212]

Iodine

Iodine (I) is a micromineral. Iodine is involved in metabolism[124,213,214] and metabolic regulation.[150,151,214,215] It is required for normal growth and development[214] and somatic growth (enhanced growth period, e.g., adolescence).[129]

Iodine is involved in neurodevelopment,[129,213] differentiation of the nerves,[214] and motor function.[129]

Iodine is involved in brain development and function,[213] cognitive function,[129] and mental development.[214] Iodine deficiency remains the most common cause of preventable mental impairment worldwide.[216]

Iodine is involved in the production of thyroid hormones[150-154] (triiodothyronine [T3] and tetraiodothyronine [T4]),[214,217] and thyroid hormone regulation.[147] It is involved in thyroid hormone regulation that ensures the energy metabolism of the cerebral cells.[147]

It is to be noted that both iodine deficiency and iodine excess may lead to thyroid dysfunction, which may manifest itself as hypothyroidism or hyperthyroidism, respectively.[214] See a qualified, accredited health practitioner if you have thyroid issues before taking iodine.

Magnesium

Magnesium (Mg) is a favourite mineral of mine and among many health professionals. Magnesium is an important mineral for normal biological function.[218] It plays an important role in all major metabolic processes[147] and metabolic function.[219] It is necessary for the functioning of over 300 enzymes in humans.[14,122,124,141,143,219-221] Magnesium is involved in DNA and RNA synthesis[14,212,220,222] and it stabilises DNA molecules and enables the maintenance of the tRNA tertiary structure[122] It is involved in the synthesis of adenosine diphosphate (ADP),[143] protein synthesis,[143,219,220] metabolism of carbohydrates, nucleic acids, and proteins,[122] transphosphorylation reactions,[212] oxidation-reduction reactions,[124,147] oxidative phosphorylation,[143,220] and nitric oxide metabolism.[136]

Magnesium is involved in ionic regulation,[147] trans-membrane ion flux,[143] ion homeostasis,[212] transmembrane electrolyte flux,[220] and participates in the transport of electrolytes through cell membranes[122] and sodium-potassium gradient across all membranes.[137] It plays a role in the control and regulation of the calcium and potassium influx at the cell membrane,[220] gating of calcium channels,[143] and the regulation of intracellular calcium levels.[137,222] Magnesium is involved in membrane structure[212] and the maintenance of cell membrane function.[137] It is a stabiliser of cell membranes.[122] It is necessary for maintaining the anatomical and functional integrity of various cellular organelles, including the mitochondria and ribosomes,[122] cytoskeletal function,[212] and maintaining normal cellular function.[222] It is involved in cell growth[141,212,219] and cell reproduction.[141,219]

Magnesium is involved in energy metabolism.[141,219,220] Magnesium is involved in ATP and ADP metabolism, via the synthesis and metabolism of ATP[14,212] and ATP-use.[212] It is an enzyme activator as part of the Mg-ATP complex,[124,143,220] the bioactive form of ATP,[143,220] along with the synthesis of ADP.[143] Magnesium is involved in glycolysis[124,143,220] and the metabolism of carbohydrates, protein, fats,[137,220] and lipids.[141] It is involved in the utilisation of intracellular energy,[137] mitochondrial health,[136] stabilisation of mitochondrial membranes,[141,219] and oxidative phosphorylation.[143,220]

Magnesium plays an important physiological role in the heart[223] and cardiovascular health. It is involved in vasomotor tone,[137,141,219,220] vascular tone,[220] maintenance of normal heart rhythm,[136,137] cardiac excitability,[141,143,219,220] nitric oxide metabolism,[136] blood pressure regulation,[141,143,219,220] blood glucose regulation,[141,143] insulin metabolism,[141,212,219,220] tyrosine kinase activity of insulin receptors,[220] and lipid metabolism.[141] Magnesium is involved in mitochondrial health,[136] stabilisation of the cell membranes of platelets and modulates their aggregation,[122] and endothelial function.[143]

Magnesium plays an important physiological role in the brain.[223] It is involved in neurotransmission,[136,141,219,220] metabolism of neurotransmitters,[136] neurotransmitter release,[220] maintenance of nerve function,[136,141,143] neuromuscular conduction,[220] and neuromuscular transmission.[137,141,218-220]

Magnesium is involved in the maintenance of normal muscle function[136,141] and plays an important physiological role in skeletal muscles.[223] It is involved in muscle contraction,[141,143,219,220] muscle relaxation,[220] neuromuscular conduction,[220] and relaxation of smooth muscle.[224] Magnesium plays a key role in mineral and bone homeostasis[122] and is essential for bone development.[122] It is involved in bone metabolism,[219] bone mineralisation,[220] bone mineral density,[219] maintenance of bone strength,[136] and bone integrity.[141]

Manganese

Manganese (Mn) is mineral that has antioxidant activity.[150,225,226] Manganese is a component of the metalloenzyme manganese superoxide dismutase (MnSOD).[21,124,225-227] It participates in enzymatic mechanisms that protect against free radicals and toxic derivatives of oxygen.[147]

Manganese is involved in energy metabolism[226] and the metabolism of carbohydrates.[225] It plays a role in energy metabolism via amino acid breakdown.[150] Manganese is involved in the metabolism of carbohydrates,[124,225] proteins,[225] and lipids.[225] Manganese is involved in the regulation of blood glucose,[226] metabolism of lipids,[225] and the metabolism of cholesterol.[124] It is involved in blood coagulation and haemostasis[226]

Manganese is involved in nerve and brain development,[225] brain physiology,[226] and cognitive functioning.[225]

Molybdenum

Molybdenum (Mo) is a micromineral. Molybdenum is an essential mineral for normal human physiology[228] and has versatile redox chemistry that is used by enzymes to catalyse diverse redox reactions.[229]

Molybdenum is an antioxidant and activator of several antioxidant enzymes that reduce lipid peroxidation.[228] For general health and liver health, manganese is involved in detoxifying excess sulphites.[230]

Research is indicating that Molybdenum has benefits in cardiometabolic health,[228,231] via glucose metabolism[231] and reducing insulin resistance.[231]

Silica

Silicon (Si) is the second most abundant element on Earth.[130,131] Silicon is rarely found in its elemental form due to its great affinity for oxygen, forming silica.[130] Silicon maintains blood vessel elasticity.[131] Silicon plays a vital role in bone health[130] bone formation,[130,232] and bone matrix quality.[232] It facilitates bone mineralisation,[232] connective tissue,[130,131] promotes the formation of collagen,[131] synthesis of elastin,[131] and glycosaminoglycans.[131,232]

Zinc

Zinc is another favourite of mine and many health professionals. Zinc is a component of around 300 enzymes[212,233] that catalyse more than 50 different physiological reactions.[233]

Zinc is involved in the maintenance of various homeostatic mechanisms,[234] enzymatic processes,[235] transcription factors,[235] synthesis of DNA and RNA,[236] metabolism of DNA and RNA,[14] DNA replication and transcription to RNA (via zinc-finger transcription factors),[237] cell growth,[234] cell proliferation,[234,236] differentiation,[236] gene transcription,[234] gene expression,[14,238,239] genomic stability,[234,239] and hormonal regulation of cell division.[234] Zinc is involved in cell structure,[236] cell membrane stabilisation,[236] provides structural stability to cell membranes,[239] cell homeostasis,[237] regulation of cell signalling,[239] intracellular signalling,[234] signal transduction,[14,234,240] redox homeostasis,[240] modulation of ion channels,[240] mitochondrial metabolism,[240] maintains metallothionein,[237,241] regulation of apoptosis,[237] and cell cycle progression.[237]

Zinc has anti-inflammatory[14,236,237,239,240,242,243] and antioxidant properties.[14,236,238,239,241,242,244,245] It is a component of superoxide dismutase (copper/zinc SOD).[241] It participates in enzymatic mechanisms that protect against free radicals and toxic derivatives of oxygen,[147] reduces oxidative stress[237,239-242,244] and free radical damage,[237,240,241] and reduces lipid peroxidation.[237,241] Zinc improves wound healing.[240]

Zinc is essential for cardiovascular health.[240] It is involved in the metabolism of lipids, carbohydrates, and protein,[212] reduction of serum total cholesterol, low-density lipoprotein (LDL) cholesterol, triglycerides, and triglyceride/high-density lipoprotein (HDL) cholesterol ratio,[212] insulin metabolism, [212] the synthesis, storage, secretion, conformational integrity, function, and action of insulin.[212]

Zinc is involved in the perception of taste.[147,237] It maintains gastrointestinal epithelial barrier function and integrity,[237,243] is involved in intestinal repair,[243] and is an essential co-enzyme for alkaline phosphatase.[246]

Zinc is involved in the optimal function of the nerves[247] and brain,[234,247] neurogenesis,[234,244] neurophysiology,[234] neurotransmission,[234,244] neuromodulation,[234] synaptic transmission,[240] signal transduction,[14] synaptic plasticity,[14] and regulation of GABA and glutamate.[245] Zinc is released during synaptic transmission, and it binds to presynaptic or postsynaptic membrane receptors.[234] Zinc plays critical roles in neuronal proliferation and differentiation, neuronal migration, and axonal growth during neurodevelopment[244]

Zinc plays a major role in immune system health.[21] It improves immunity[240] via the development and function of cells mediating innate immunity[236,243] and regulation of the innate and adaptive immune responses.[236] Zinc supports a Th1 cytokine-mediated immune response[162] and is important for the intracellular binding of tyrosine kinase to T-cell receptors.[246]

Coenzyme Q10

Coenzyme Q10 has 2 forms, Ubiquinol (reduced form) and Ubiquinone (oxidised form). Ubiquinol is considered the superior form of Coenzyme Q10, as it is readily active[248] and has greater bioavailability.[249] Coenzyme Q10 is involved in energy metabolism[250] and mitochondrial energetics.[251-253] It is an essential carrier of electrons in mitochondrial oxidative phosphorylation for ATP synthesis.[248] It improves exercise capacity.[254]

Coenzyme Q10 has anti-inflammatory[250,253,255] and antioxidant[248-253,255,256] properties. It works as an antioxidant in the cytosol by trapping peroxyl radicals that mediate lipid peroxidation.[248] As an antioxidant, ubiquinol (along with glutathione) plays an essential role in reducing phospholipid peroxidation and ferroptosis.[248] Coenzyme Q10 reduces oxidative stress[248] and inflammation.[255]

Glutathione

Glutathione is commonly known as "the master antioxidant".[70] This biological antioxidant is found in nearly all mammalian tissues,[70] especially in the cytoplasm and mitochondria,[257] and is the most prevalent non-protein intracellular thiol.[70] It plays a crucial role in various vital aspects of cellular homeostasis.[70] Similar to many selenoenzymes, it contains one redox-sensitive selenocysteine amino acid that plays a crucial role in the enzymatic reduction of hydrogen peroxide[257,258] (to water)[258] and soluble lipid hydroperoxides.[257] Glutathione has antioxidant[70,257-260] and anti-inflammatory[259] properties. Glutathione serves as the source of reducing equivalents essential for its activity. As an antioxidant enzyme, glutathione peroxidase regulates the equilibrium between beneficial and detrimental levels of reactive oxygen species.[257] Glutathione is involved in the transport of amino acids,[260] acts as a coenzyme for enzymes,[260] and protects against oxygen radicals and toxic compounds.[260] It is involved in numerous significant detoxification processes and possesses a remarkable ability to prevent cellular damage caused by oxidative stress.[70] Consequently, the intracellular redox state, which is defined by the levels and ratio of oxidised (GSSG) to reduced (GSH) glutathione, is regarded as a key indicator of cellular health.[70]

Lipoic acid

Lipoic acid is involved in the metabolism of proteins, carbohydrates, glucose, and fats.[241] It acts as an essential cofactor for mitochondrial enzymes.[261-263]

Lipoic acid is an antioxidant[261-263] and endogenous thiol antioxidant.[182,241] It regenerates antioxidants, such as glutathione, vitamin C, and vitamin E,[182] and increases the effectiveness of other antioxidants, such as glutathione.[263,264] Lipoic acid quenches reactive oxygen species and reduces oxidative stress and free radical damage.[182] A use and clinical application is oxidative stress.[182,241] It can chelate metals, such as cadmium, copper, iron and mercury.[182]

Lutein

Lutein is an antioxidant[265] and potent free radical scavenger.[266] In skin health, Lutein protects the skin from ultraviolet radiation-associated oxidation and inflammation.[266]

Lutein promotes vascular health[266] and reduces the damage of blood vessels by decreasing the amount of oxidised low-density lipoproteins (LDL).[266] Lutein can slow down the progression of age-related macular degeneration[265,266] and cataracts.[266]

Omega-3

Omega-3 is a polyunsaturated fatty acid. Omega-3 is involved in cell membrane phospholipid composition.[267-269] It is involved in the improvement of cell membrane function,[268,270] cell membrane fluidity,[269,270] composition of lipid rafts,[270] cell signalling,[271] act as messenger molecules,[270] regulation of ion transport through membranes,[270] eicosanoid metabolism,[267-269] and gene expression.[269] Research has shown an association between omega-3 fatty acid consumption and telomere length.[270]

Omega-3 has anti-inflammatory[87,268-274] and antioxidant[270,274] properties, modulates oxidative stress,[270,274] and modulates neuroinflammation.[269] The uses and clinical applications include inflammation.[268] Omega-3 decreases inflammation via protectins and resolvins, which decrease neutrophil and T-cell recruitment and reduce inflammation in atherosclerosis,[273] potentially having a protective role.

In cardiometabolic health, Omega-3 decreases platelet activation and aggregation,[271-273,275] reduces fibrin generation, velocity of fibrin polymerisation, and peak thrombin generated,[276] reduces P-selectin expression,[272] improves lipid profiles,[267,268,273] including reduction of triglycerides[271,273] and very low-density lipoprotein (VLDL),[271] lowers blood pressure.[271] It is involved in vascular relaxation[272] endothelial function,[271,273] and improving cardiometabolic profile in women with polycystic ovary syndrome (PCOS)[277]

Omega-3 has been found to increase synaptic development and functionality,[269] have effects on synaptic integrity and plasticity.[269] It modulates the release of neurotransmitters, myelination, and neuronal growth,[269] and is involved in signal transduction in the nervous system.[270] DHA and arachidonic acid are the most important polyunsaturated acids in the brain.[269] DHA is one of the major building structures of membrane phospholipids of the brain[278] and DHA is necessary for neuronal function.[278] Uses and clinical applications include altered composition of brain cell membranes, neurones, oligodendrocytes and astrocytes,[278] altered composition of myelin, nerve endings (synaptosomes) and mitochondria,[278] neurosensory imbalance,[278] and neurodegenerative disorders,[269] such as Alzheimer's disease and Parkinson's disease.[269]

Omega-11

Fatty fish species generally serve as excellent sources of the beneficial omega-3 fatty acids EPA (20:5n-3) and DHA (22:6n-3) for human consumption.[279] Nonetheless, variations exist in the fatty acid profiles among pelagic fish species. For instance, North Atlantic fish such as capelin and herring exhibit lower concentrations of EPA and DHA compared to the South American sardine, with levels around 8% versus approximately 23% of total fatty acids, respectively.[279] Conversely, these North Atlantic species are more abundant in long-chain (LC) MUFA, particularly cetoleic acid (22:1n-11), which constitutes about 17-22% compared to roughly 1% found in sardines.[279]

Research indicates that cetoleic acid stimulates the synthesis of EPA and DHA from ALA (alpha linoleic acid).[279] Additionally, research shows that fish oil containing cetoleic acid increases the Omega-3 index.[280,281]

CET03® is a fish oil product derived from North Atlantic herring and contains around 20% of omega-3 polyunsaturated fatty acids combined with 50% monounsaturated fatty acids, including around 23% cetoleic acid (C 22:1 *n*-11). Research indicates that there is a metabolic transformation of 18:3 n-3 (ALA) into EPA and DHA in step with the intake of cetoleic acid.[280] A 12-week double-blind randomised intervention trial with a parallel group design was conducted to investigate the effect of CET03® versus fish oil on omega-3 status. The participants consumed either two 1 g capsules of CET03® daily or two 1 g fish oil capsules daily with food. Each CETO3® herring capsule contained 200 mg of DHA/EPA (i.e., 400 mg per day), whereas each fish oil capsule contained 300 mg DHA/EPA (i.e., 600 mg per day). After 12 weeks, the study demonstrated that CET03® (containing a lower dose of omega-3) increased the Omega-3 Index (4.96% to 5.73%, 15.52% increase), comparable to Fish oil (5.55% to 6.24%, 12.43% increase). Compared to the fish oil capsules used in this trial, it would appear from the results of this pilot study, on a pro-rata dose equivalence, that CET03® might deliver a 50% improvement in the Omega-3 Index.

Two intervention studies were conducted as part of this pilot study, both designed as randomised, double-blind, placebo-controlled trials.[281] The CetoIndex study assessed the omega-3 index utilising a blood spot collection kit (Omegaquant). Meanwhile, the Optihud study evaluated skin quality parameters in healthy women through the VISIA system. The cetoleic-rich oil was sourced from North Atlantic fish and was characterised by a high concentration of long-chain mono-unsaturated fatty acids, notably cetoleic acid (C22:1 n-11) and gondoic acid (C20:1 n-9). In the CetoIndex placebo-controlled study, the omega-3 index exhibited an increase comparable to that observed with fish oil that contains elevated levels of omega-3 fatty acids. In the Optihud placebo-controlled study, the cetoleic-rich oil was found to diminish erythema in the skin, which serves as an indicator of inflammation. The findings from this pilot study endorse the application of cetoleic-rich oil for enhancing the omega-3 index, with potential advantages for skin inflammation.[281]

Resveratrol

Resveratrol is a naturally occurring polyphenolic compound.[282] Resveratrol activates the energy sensor AMP-activated protein kinase (AMPK), which in turn stimulates NAD^+ (re)synthesis.[72] Resveratrol exhibits a variety of functions, including antioxidant[283,284] and anti-inflammatory effects,[285,286] reduces pro-inflammatory cytokines,[285] cardiovascular protection,[286] lowers total cholesterol,[282,287] lowers systolic blood pressure,[282,287] reduces glycated haemoglobin (HbA1c),[282] increases cerebral blood flow during task performance,[283] neuroprotection,[286] and anti-ageing benefits.[284,286]

As an antioxidant, resveratrol is known for its role as a scavenger of reactive oxygen species (ROS) such as hydroxyl-induced, superoxide-induced, and metal-induced radicals.[284] The mechanisms through which resveratrol contributes to anti-ageing primarily involve the reduction of oxidative stress, alleviation of inflammatory responses, enhancement of mitochondrial function, and regulation of apoptosis.[286] In clinical studies, resveratrol has been shown to moderately reduce systolic blood pressure in individuals with hypertension, as well as lower blood glucose levels in patients with type 2 diabetes.[284]

In an animal study, Resveratrol was found to activate SIRT3 either directly or indirectly, which resulted in a decrease in the acetylation of the mitochondrial transcription factor A (TFAM), thereby alleviating mitochondrial dysfunction in the hearts of diabetic subjects.[76]

Carnitine

Carnitine is an amino acid. Carnitine plays an essential role in cellular energy metabolism,[288] metabolism of fatty acids,[289] and is necessary to deliver long-chain fatty acids from the cytosol into the mitochondrial matrix.[290]

Carnitine has anti-inflammatory,[290] antioxidant,[290] cardioprotective effects,[290] and neuroprotective functions.[290] Carnitine improves cardiac energy metabolism,[290] attention concentration,[291] and physical and mental fatigue.[288,291] Carnitine has been found to reduce total cholesterol[288] and fat mass[288] and increase muscle mass.[288] Additionally, research has found amelioration of muscle soreness and improved muscle damage biomarkers.[290]

Creatine

I have been prescribing creatine for various physical, mental, and cognitive health benefits since 1998. Creatine is synthesised endogenously, mainly in the kidneys,[292-294] liver,[292-294] pancreas,[292,293] and brain,[292,294] through a two-step process that utilises three amino acids: arginine, glycine, and methionine.[292,293] Creatine can be consumed via dietary sources such as seafood, red meat, and poultry, as well as through supplementation.[293] Once creatine enters the bloodstream, around 95% is retained in skeletal muscle, with roughly 67% being transformed into phosphocreatine and about 33% remaining as free creatine.[293] Phosphocreatine interacts with adenosine diphosphate (ADP) and is broken down by creatine kinase to regenerate adenosine triphosphate (ATP).[292,293] Interestingly, creatine has some ability to cross the blood-brain barrier through microcapillary endothelial cells that express the creatine transporter SLC6A8,[292,295] leading to its accumulation in the brain.[292] The supplementation of creatine enhances the levels of muscle creatine and phosphocreatine (PCr), as demonstrated through both nuclear magnetic resonance (NMR) spectroscopy and muscle biopsy analyses.[292] Creatine is important for energy metabolism.[294]

Creatine is an effective ergogenic aid to improve sports performance,[292] enhance resistance training,[293] enhance resistance training adaptations,[293] enhance adaptation to exercise training,[292] improve performance in a single bout of intense exercise,[293] improve intense, short-duration, intermittent performance,[293] improve resistance to fatigue,[292] and increase power output.[293]

Creatine increases time to exhaustion during high-intensity endurance activities,[293] increases anaerobic work capacity and performance,[293] increases muscle efficiency,[293] increases muscle function,[292] increases muscle mass,[292] improves buffering capacity,[293] augments glycogen resynthesis,[293] resynthesising adenosine triphosphate (ATP),[292] enhances ATP transport,[293] and positively effects neuromuscular activity.[293]

Some of the additional functions of creatine are anti-inflammatory,[293] antioxidant,[293] lowers oxidative stress,[293] enhances physical peak performance,[295] improves cognitive function[292] and cognition,[296] improves cognitive performance,[295] improves cognitive performance of elderly people,[297] improves cognitive processing speed,[295] improves memory,[292,294] long-term memory,[297] and recall,[292] improves working memory,[292] increases body mass,[293] increases mitochondria biogenesis,[293] and improves the performance of activities of daily living.[298] Regarding increases in body mass, this phenomenon may be linked to short-term creatine loading, which affects intracellular and/or total body water retention, ultimately resulting in an increase in body mass.[293] Creatine may have benefits in neurodegenerative diseases[292,295] (such as amyotrophic lateral sclerosis, Duchenne muscular dystrophy, Parkinson's disease[292]) via reducing oxidative stress and mitochondrial damage, and improving energy metabolism,[292] and in mental health (for example, depression, anxiety, post-traumatic brain disorder).[292] Additionally, creatine has potential in people suffering from concussion and traumatic brain injury.[292]

A double-blind, randomised, prospective study featuring a balanced cross-over design demonstrated the impact of a high dose of creatine (on one night, 0.35 g/kg of creatine was administered, while on the other night, 0.35 g/kg of placebo was given).[295] The findings indicated that creatine enhanced cognitive performance that was impaired due to sleep deprivation, with effects persisting for up to 9 hours and peaking at 4 hours post-oral administration.[295]

Intramuscular levels of creatine can be enhanced further when the intake of creatine monohydrate is paired with exercise, carbohydrates, a combination of carbohydrates and protein, or lipoic acid.[292] Additionally, when creatine is taken with carbohydrates, creatine improves the replenishment of glycogen and glycogen levels.[293] Research has indicated that creatine was associated to a reduction in the length of post-traumatic amnesia, intubation periods, and hospital stays. It has also been shown to enhance neurophysical, cognitive, personality/behavioural, and social dimensions, as well as to alleviate post-traumatic headaches, dizziness, and fatigue.[292]

Glutamine

Glutamine is one of my favourite amino acids and it is a favourite among health professionals. Glutamine is involved in protein synthesis,[299,300] cell proliferation,[301] cell integrity,[300,302] extracellular matrix synthesis,[300] signal transduction,[299,300,302] cell signalling,[300] neurotransmission,[300] activating intracellular signalling pathways,[299,300,302] and pH homeostasis.[303] Glutamine enhances intestinal and whole-body growth[304] and protects cells against apoptosis and cellular stresses during normal and pathologic conditions.[305] Glutamine has anti-inflammatory effects,[300] suppresses pro-inflammatory signalling pathways,[305] has redox potential,[300] and is an essential precursor for the antioxidant glutathione peroxidase.[299] It is involved in energy metabolism[301] gluconeogenesis,[300] and glycogenesis (formation of glycogen).[301]

Glutamine is an essential nutrient for small intestine function and is involved in liver health.[300] It enhances intestinal and whole-body growth,[304] promotes enterocyte proliferation,[304,305] regulates tight junction proteins,[305] tight junction stabilisation,[300] regulates intestinal barrier function in injury and infection,[304] and enhances ion transport by the digestive system.[304]

Glutamine is involved in immune function,[300] is essential for lymphocyte proliferation,[303,306] cytokine production,[303] neutrophil bacterial killing activity,[303] and macrophage activation and phagocytosis plus secretory activities.[303]

Theanine

L-theanine is a non-protein water-soluble amino acid that is characteristically found in tea plants,[307-309] particularly green tea (*Camellia sinensis*).[307,308,310-312] L-theanine has anti-inflammatory,[309,313] antioxidant,[309,313] cardiovascular protection,[313] neuroprotective,[313] anxiolytic (anti-anxiety),[313] calming,[313] metabolic regulation,[313] and immune-regulating properties.[313] Additionally, theanine has been reported to improve sleep latency and[308] sleep disturbance.

Research on L-theanine has reported improvements in cognitive function,[308,311] including learning and memory,[307] depression,[308,311] anxiety,[308,310,311,314] stress,[314] and sleep.[308,311] L-theanine has been found to elicit changes in alpha brain wave activity with concurrent increases in selective attention during the execution of mental tasks.[307]

Collagen

Collagen products have been popular for the last few decades, particularly for skin health. In the skin, collagen, elastic fibres, and hyaluronic acid are major structural constituents of the dermal extracellular matrix.[315] Research shows that collagen improves skin hydration,[315-317] skin elasticity,[315-317] wrinkle reduction,[315,317] dermal collagen density,[316] skin ageing,[316,317] and wound healing.[316] Additionally, hydrolysed collagen may contain biologically active peptides that are able to reach joint tissues and exert chondroprotective effects.[318]

A systematic review and meta-analysis investigated the effects of hydrolysed collagen supplementation on human skin, focusing on the process of skin ageing.[317] In the meta-analysis, a grouped analysis of various studies indicated positive outcomes of hydrolysed collagen supplementation in comparison to placebo regarding skin hydration, elasticity, and wrinkle reduction. The results demonstrating enhanced hydration and elasticity were further validated in the subgroup meta-analysis. According to the findings, the consumption of hydrolysed collagen over a period of 90 days was found to be effective in reducing skin ageing, as it reduced wrinkles and enhanced both skin elasticity and hydration.[317]

A randomised, double-blind, placebo-controlled trial examined the impact of low-molecular-weight collagen peptide (1,000 mg daily) on skin hydration, wrinkling, and elasticity in women aged 40 to 60 years.[315] After 12 weeks, there were significant improvements in the condition of photoaged skin, with significant improvements in skin hydration observed as early as 6 weeks into the treatment, and enhancements in skin wrinkling and elasticity noted after 12 weeks of supplementation.[315]

A meta-analysis of randomised placebo-controlled trials indicated that collagen treatment resulted in a notable reduction in the total Western Ontario and McMaster Universities Osteoarthritis Index (WOMAC) index score.[319] Following a subgroup analysis of the WOMAC subscores, collagen supplementation demonstrated a significant reduction in the stiffness subscore. The findings of this meta-analysis suggest that collagen is effective in alleviating osteoarthritis symptoms through the reduction of both the total WOMAC index and the Visual Analog Scale (VAS) score.[319]

UC-II

UC-II is an undenatured type II collagen.[320-322] The proposed mechanism of action for UC-II involves the induction and migration of T regulatory cells (Tregs) to sites of inflammation and damage.[323] Additionally, the role of Tregs may be significant in moderating symptoms of osteoarthritis, as in vitro research has demonstrated that Tregs secrete anti-inflammatory cytokines that encourage chondrocytes to produce components of the cartilage matrix.[323] Native collagen possesses a distinct immune-mediated mechanism that necessitates the identification and recognition of its epitopes to suppress inflammation and tissue degradation at the joint level.[318]

A randomised, double-blind, placebo-controlled study investigated the effect of UC-II on knee joint function in healthy individuals.[324] After 120 days of supplementation, participants in the UC-II® group showed a statistically significant improvement compared to the placebo group in Knee Injury and Osteoarthritis Outcome Score (KOOS) metrics, including reduced pain while standing upright and while ascending or descending stairs, as well as reduced discomfort when climbing stairs, bending down to retrieve an object, or squatting during periods of intense physical activity ($p<0.05$).[324]

A randomised, double-blind, placebo-controlled study investigated the effect of UC-II 40 mg versus placebo for 120 days on knee joint function.[320] The participants in the UC-II group showed statistically significantly greater increase in the ability to extend the knee at day 120 as compared to the placebo group ($81.0 \pm 1.3^{\circ}$ vs $74.0 \pm 2.2^{\circ}$, $p = 0.011$). It was also noted that the participants in the UC-II group exercised longer before experiencing any initial joint discomfort at day 120 (2.8 ± 0.5 minutes, $p = 0.019$), compared to baseline (1.4 ± 0.2 minutes).[320]

A randomised, double-blind, placebo-controlled study assessed the effect of undenatured collagen on knee flexibility in healthy subjects who experience activity-related joint discomfort.[325] After 24 weeks, the group receiving UC-II supplementation exhibited a statistically significant mean increase of 3.23° in range of motion flexion, in contrast to the mean increase of 0.21° observed in the placebo group. A notable difference in active range of motion flexion between the UC-II group and the placebo group was observed as early as week 8 of supplementation, and this improvement continued to be significant throughout the duration of the study.[325] Additionally, there was an increase in knee range of motion extension of 2.21° was recorded over time in the UC-II group ($p = 0.0061$), whereas the placebo group exhibited a non-significant increase of 1.27° ($p > 0.05$).[325]

A randomised clinical trial evaluated the safety and efficacy of UC-II 40 mg compared to a combination of glucosamine hydrochloride 1,500 mg and chondroitin sulfate 1,200 mg in the treatment of osteoarthritis of the knee.[322] After 90 days, participants taking UC-II found improvements in pain walking on flat surface, difficulty walking on a flat surface, pain during climbing up and down stairs, night pain, resting pain, and performing heavy domestic duties. UC-II was significantly better than Glucosamine and Chondroitin for ascending stairs at 30 days and 60 days, at night while in bed, pain during climbing up and down stairs at 90 days, and difficulty walking on a flat surface at 90 days. Additionally, there was a significant improvement in pain when getting up from a sitting position.

A multicentre randomised, double-blind, placebo-controlled study investigated the effect of UC-II 40 mg, Glucosamine hydrochloride 1,500 mg and Chondroitin sulfate 1,200 mg, or placebo on moderate to severe osteoarthritis of the knee.[323] After 180 days, the UC-II group showed reductions in pain and stiffness and improvements in physical function compared to placebo. When compared against Glucosamine and Chondroitin, UC-II showed reductions in pain and stiffness.[323]

Urolithin A

Urolithin A is a naturally occurring compound (postbiotic) produced by gut microbiota from consumed ellagitannins and ellagic acid, which are complex polyphenols found in foods like pomegranate,[78,326,327] berries,[78,327] strawberries,[326] raspberries,[326] nuts,[326,327] and walnuts.[78] Urolithin A has been shown to increase mitochondrial health,[78,326] mitochondrial function,[328] mitochondrial efficiency,[78] mitophagy,[78,326,328] increase skeletal muscle function,[326] improve muscle function,[78,328] improve muscle strength,[78,326,328] increase leg muscle strength,[78] improved muscle endurance,[328] increase muscle performance,[78] increase exercise performance,[78] increase physical performance,[78] aerobic endurance (peak oxygen consumption [VO_2]),[78] decrease inflammation,[326,328] neuroprotective effects,[326] and has the potential to improve healthy ageing[326] and lifespan.[326] Urolithin A enhanced the synthesis of proteoglycan and collagen, which are essential components of the extracellular matrix.[326]

Urolithin A has been shown to enhance mitochondrial health.[326] This advantage is facilitated by the removal and recycling of dysfunctional mitochondria through a selective autophagy mechanism known as mitophagy.[326] Mitophagy becomes compromised with advancing age and in various age-associated diseases. Restoring appropriate levels of mitophagy presents a promising approach to mitigate the age-related deterioration of organ function.[326]

Potential herbal combinations with NMN

NMN can be used as a standalone active ingredient or in conjunction with herbs. If you're considering taking NMN alongside other products, it's important to reflect on the results you aim to achieve and the underlying mechanisms of action. Some potential benefits include enhanced energy levels, improved immune system function, better cardiovascular health, increased aerobic capacity, and greater longevity.

When creating and formulating products that incorporate NMN along with herbs, keep in mind the mechanisms of action and the synergy between NMN and the proposed herbs. Utilise your knowledge of nutritional biochemistry, anatomy, physiology, and pathophysiology to guide you in developing a product that meets your desired outcomes.

Herbal medicines have been used for thousands of years for the prevention and management of various health conditions, particularly chronic disease.[22-24] The World Health Organization (WHO) estimates that approximately 80% of the world's population use traditional medicine for their primary health care needs and most of this therapy involves the use of plant extracts or the active components from plants.[329] Plants have been used for healing purposes throughout human history, and form the origin of modern medicine.[329,330] Modern Western herbal medicine emphasises the effects of herbs on the whole body and individual body systems. The aim of herbal medicine is to produce persisting improvements in health and wellbeing. Herbal medicine practitioners aim to treat the underlying risk factors and triggers of disease and may prescribe herbs, singly or in combination with other herbal medicines as a formula, aimed at correcting patterns of dysfunction rather than targeting the presenting symptoms.[24] Herbs support the body's natural processes and flow. Herbs may be chosen and utilised for their adaptogen,[25] analgesic,[27] anti-inflammatory,[26-29] antioxidant,[27-30] antiplatelet,[331] antispasmodic,[31,32] anxiolytic,[31-33] carminative,[332] cognitive,[333,334] digestive,[332] expectorant,[335] hepatoprotective,[34-36] hypoglycaemic,[35] immunomodulatory,[27-29] insulin sensitivity,[336,337] nervine,[338] nerve tonic,[37,38] neuroprotective[26] sedative,[32,33,339] tonic,[332] vasodilatory,[340] or wound healing[341,342] properties. Please be aware of any allergies and potential interactions with medications. It should be noted that it is always best for herbal medicines to be prescribed by a qualified naturopath, herbalist, or health professional with theoretical and clinical training in herbal medicine. Herbs are not to be prescribed, suggested, taken, or used during pregnancy or breastfeeding without consulting a health professional. This section provides a summary of various herbal medicines that could potentially be taken alongside NMN or be combined in formulations with NMN.

Ashwagandha

Ashwagandha (*Withania somnifera*) (root) is one of my most favourite herbs. I first learned about Ashwagandha in 1996 and attended a two-day conference on Chinese and Ayurvedic herbs (where Ashwagandha was a major feature) in early 1997, which strengthened my love for this herb. The name "Ashwagandha" originates from the word "ashwa", signifying horse. It is thought that by ingesting the root, individuals acquire the strength, power, and abilities akin to those of a horse. The latter portion of the name, "gandha", denotes fragrance and alludes to the distinct scent of the plant's fresh root.[28] The root is mainly used in therapeutics, along with some combinations of root and leaves.[27] Ashwagandha is known as the "rejuvenator" and "revitaliser".[30,343] It has long been used in traditional Ayurvedic medicine to enhance memory and improve cognition.[344] There has been a growing interest in the potential health benefits of Ashwagandha, particularly in the areas of stress management, cognitive function, and physical performance.[28] Some of the actions and uses of Ashwagandha include adaptogen (adapting the body to stress),[26-29,345] reducing stress,[26-28,345] reducing serum cortisol levels,[26] anxiety,[27-29,345,346] depression,[29,345] general weakness,[345] and strengthens the nervous system,[28] and has neuroprotective action.[26]

Ashwagandha is used for improving memory,[29,344] cognition,[28,344] having nootropic effects,[27] concentration,[29] attention,[344] improving information processing speed,[344] mood,[29] insomnia,[29] endurance and stamina,[343] and cardiorespiratory endurance and stamina.[343] Ashwagandha has tonic,[28] anti-inflammatory,[26-29] antioxidant,[27-30] cardioprotective,[345] immune modulating,[27-29,345] antibacterial,[27,28] hepatoprotective,[27] neuroprotective,[28] sleep-promoting[345],[29] and analgesic[27] properties. Ashwagandha enhances general wellbeing,[26] and impacts improvements in upper and lower-body strength,[30] enhancing cardiorespiratory endurance and improving quality of life in healthy athletic adults.[343]

Ashwagandha and Okra

A randomised, double-blind, placebo-controlled trial was conducted to provide proof-of-concept for assessing the effectiveness and tolerability of a proprietary mixture of standardised extracts from Ashwagandha (*Withania somnifera*) root and Okra (*Hibiscus esculentus*/*Abelmoschus esculentus*) fruit (digexin®) in alleviating constipation and enhancing the quality of life in adults.[345] The participants were randomised into Active 300 mg, Active 500 mg, or placebo for 14 days. At the conclusion of the 2-week study, participants receiving digexin® exhibited a decrease in diarrhoea, constipation, indigestion, and reflux discomfort. They had improvements in complete spontaneous bowel movements and overall bowel performance, alongside a reduction in stress levels. Furthermore, there were notable improvements in physical function and energy, as well as sleep quality, which included factors such as awakening from sleep, behaviour after waking, and the ability to fall asleep. Additionally, there were significant increases in serum serotonin, gastrin, and interleukin-10, while levels of interleukin-6 and cortisol decreased. Participants reported reduced physical discomfort, psychosocial discomfort, dissatisfaction, and a decrease in worries and concerns.[345]

A randomised, double-blind, placebo-controlled study was conducted to re-evaluate the efficacy and tolerability of digexin® (Ashwagandha (*Withania somnifera*) root and Okra (*Hibiscus esculentus*/*Abelmoschus esculentus*) fruit) in alleviating gastrointestinal distress and associated gastrointestinal factors in a larger number of subjects with functional constipation supplemented over an extended period. Participants were randomly assigned to receive Active 300 mg, Active 500 mg, or a placebo for 60 days.[347] At the conclusion of the 2-

month study, participants in the digexin® group exhibited a decrease in abdominal pain, constipation, diarrhea, indigestion, and reflux. Additionally, there was a reduction in gastrointestinal transit time, an improvement in complete spontaneous bowel movements and overall bowel performance, and an improvement in intestinal integrity as indicated by lower serum zonulin levels. Furthermore, sleep quality improved, as evidenced by fewer nighttime awakenings, better behaviour after waking, and an easier time falling asleep. The study also noted improved inflammatory modulation, characterised by decreased serum IL-6 and increased IL-10 levels. Participants showed elevated serum levels of gastrin and serotonin, a reduction in serum cortisol, and lower scores for depression and anxiety. Overall, there was a notable decrease in physical discomfort, psychosocial distress, dissatisfaction, and various worries and concerns.[347]

Berberine

I have been prescribing berberine-containing herbs since the beginning of my career. Berberine has increased in popularity over the last few years. Various studies have reported the traditional uses Berberis plants for the treatment of cardiometabolic conditions.[348] Berberis species contain various bioactive compounds, such as alkaloids, polyphenols, flavonoids, and anthocyanins.[348] Berberine is one of the most commonly reported alkaloids from various Berberis species,[336,348-350] including *Berberis aristata* and *Berberis vulgaris*. Berberine is mostly found in Berberis sp. root bark, root, and stem bark.[348]

Some of the actions of Berberine include reducing fasting blood glucose,[349,350] 2-hour postprandial blood glucose,[350] glycosylated haemoglobin ($HbA1_c$),[336,349] insulin resistance,[336,350] triglyceride level,[337,349-351] total cholesterol,[336,349-351] low-density lipoprotein cholesterol (LDL-cholesterol),[336,349,351] systolic blood pressure,[337] inflammation,[336,350] high-sensitivity-C reactive protein (hs-CRP),[350] interleukin-6 (IL-6),[350] tumour necrosis factor-α (TNF-α),[350] and waist circumference in females.[337]

Berberine has been found to increase glycolysis,[336] insulin secretion,[336] and insulin sensitivity.[336,337] Some of the applications of Berberine include cardiometabolic syndrome,[336,337,350] insulin resistance,[336,350] and inflammation,[350] Berberine may also reduce the risk of developing cardiometabolic syndrome through its beneficial effects on the gut microbiota.[336] Composition of the gut microbiota affects cardiometabolic health.[336] This is interesting as we learn more and more about the microbiome and its effects on health.

Brahmi

Brahmi (*Bacopa monnieri*) (whole plant) is another one of my favourite herbs. I have been prescribing Brahmi to patients for over 26 years. The name Brahmi is derived from the word "Brama", the mythical "creator" in the Hindu pantheon.[352] Brahmi has been used for thousands of years in Ayurvedic medicine,[352,353] either alone or in combination with other herbs, as an enhancer of cognitive performance.[353] Among various medicinal Ayurvedic herbs, *Bacopa monnieri* is considered a herb of grace.[38] Brahmi was traditionally used as a restorative in debilitated conditions.[352] Brahmi contains bacosides, alkaloids, glycosides, sterol glycosides, saponins, and flavonoids.[38] Bacosides play essential roles in neuronal health with Bacosides A and B being responsible for most neuropharmacological and nootropic effects.[38]

Some of the actions and uses of Brahmi include cognitive effects,[38,354] memory-enhancing effects,[338,352,354,355] recall,[353] enhanced cognitive performance[338,353,356] and learning,[352,355] improved speed of visual information processing, learning rate, and memory consolidation,[357] improvement in auditory-visual learning[355] improvement in speed of attention,[356] reduction of acetylcholinesterase activity,[37] increased cerebral blood flow,[37] reducing anxiety,[352] and analgesic,[352] anti-inflammatory[338,352] and antioxidant[37,38] effects. Brahmi is a major nootropic herb.[38,352,354] Brahmi is a nervine (anti-stress effects),[338] adaptogen,[358] nerve tonic,[37,38] and calming[352] herb that reduces anxiety.[338,346,355]

Chaste tree

Chaste tree (*Vitex agnus-castus*) (berry) is a small tree or shrub native to European, Mediterranean, and Central Asian countries.[359] Chaste tree is commonly used for the management of female reproductive disorders, notably premenstrual syndrome (PMS),[360-364] menstrual disorders (such as amenorrhoea and dysmenorrhoea),[363] cyclical mastalgia,[363,364] corpus luteum insufficiency,[363] hyperprolactinemia,[363] infertility,[360-363] and menopause.[363].

Chaste tree is widely used for its ability to regulate hormonal balance and improve the oestrogen-to-progesterone ratio; an imbalance that is implicated in endometriosis.[365-367] Vitex agnus-castus may affect hormones and medicines such as oral contraceptives. Consult your health professional before use.

Dong Quai

Dong quai (*Angelica polymorpha*) root has been used for thousands of years in traditional Chinese, Korean and Japanese medicines.[368] Dong Quai has been likened to the "female ginseng".[368] It is traditionally used to support circulation and immune function, and for female health,[80] gynaecological conditions,[368] and menstrual health.[80] Dong quai is used for the treatment of menstrual cramping, irregular menstruation, and menopausal symptoms.[369]

Echinacea

Echinacea (*Echinacea purpurea*) has been traditionally used to improve the immune system,[370] for wound healing,[370] respiratory symptoms caused by bacterial infections,[370] respiratory conditions,[371] bronchitis,[372] infections,[372] ulcers,[372] skin disorders,[372] inflammation,[371] and wounds.[372] It is used to treat the common cold.[372,373] Echinacea has antimicrobial,[370-372] immunomodulatory,[371,372] and anti-inflammatory[370,371] properties.

Ginkgo

Ginkgo (*Ginkgo biloba*) (leaf) use has a long history and is one of the most widely used herbal medicines in Europe and the US.[374] It is one of my favourite herbs for cognitive function and memory. Ginkgo is used to improve memory[375,376] and concentration.[375] Ginkgo has numerous actions, including antioxidant,[374,376] free radical scavenging,[374] anti-inflammatory,[376] antiplatelet[377] effects, along with reducing platelet activating factor,[374] modifying membrane fluidity,[374] signal transduction,[374] and mitochondrial protection.[378]

Ginkgo has been found to increase blood flow[379] and circulation,[379] improve vasodilation,[378] decrease blood viscosity,[378] and enhance microperfusion.[378] Ginkgolides, one of the active components of Ginkgo, are potent inhibitors of platelet activating factor.[380] A 20-year follow-up study found that those taking Ginkgo (EGb761®) declined less rapidly (as assessed via Mini-Mental State Examination, a test for cognitive impairment, such as problems with thinking, communication, understanding and memory), whereas the Piracetam group declined more rapidly.[378]

Gotu Kola

Centella asiatica (Gotu Kola) (leaf; whole plant) has been used as a medicinal plant since ancient times for a wide range of indications.[381-384] Gotu Kola has cognitive,[382,385-387] antioxidant,[381,382,386] lipid peroxidation reduction,[381,386] anti-inflammatory,[382] neuroprotective,[383] nervine tonic,[382] and microcirculation[382] properties.

The applications of Gotu Kola include memory,[386] cognition,[382,385-387] stress,[387] generalised anxiety disorder,[387,388] depression,[387] various neurological disorders,[387] nervous system disorders,[383] sleep issues,[383] venous insufficiency,[382-384] varicose ulcers,[382] striae gravidarum (stretch marks),[382,384] skin disorders,[383] eczema,[382] psoriasis,[382] gastrointestinal disorders,[383] and for wound healing.[382-384,386]

Korean Ginseng

I have been prescribing Korean Ginseng (*Panax ginseng*) root to patients for over 26 years for its numerous actions as an adaptogen, enhancing cognition, and increasing energy levels. Korean Ginseng is a traditional herbal medicine that has been used therapeutically for more than 2,000 years. The name panax refers to "all healing", and this possibly originates from the traditional belief that ginseng acts as a panacea and heals all aspects of illness.[389] Panax ginseng has a longstanding history in Chinese medicine as a herb for enhancing energy levels and for reinforcing vital energy.[390]

From a traditional Chinese medicine perspective, Panax ginseng is considered to contribute to the enhancement and invigoration of vital energy by effectively tonifying the Qi associated with the spleen, lungs, heart, and kidneys.[390] In addition, Qi is instrumental in the production of blood. Panax ginseng facilitates the body's blood production, promotes the smoothness of blood vessels, and aids in the restoration of both Qi and blood, thereby nourishing the heart and soothing the mind through the tonification of Qi.[390]

Research has shown that Korean Ginseng enhances cognitive performance,[391] has favourable effects on cognition in young healthy people,[392] improves scores on a secondary memory, which is a composite of memory tasks,[392] and improves fatigue in people with chronic fatigue.[391] A study found that Korean Ginseng improved cognitive performance and subjective feelings of mental fatigue during sustained mental activity.[393]

Panax ginseng has adaptogenic,[358] neuroprotective,[390] anti-depressant,[390] tonic,[390] regulating the function of HPA axis,[390] antiplatelet,[389,394] vasorelaxant,[389] antioxidant,[389-391] anti-inflammatory,[389,390] immune modulation,[390,391] and anti-ageing[390] properties, in addition to improving blood circulation and lipid profile.[389] As Korean Ginseng is a stimulating adaptogen, generally it is best taken in the first half of the day.

Lemon Balm

Lemon Balm (*Melissa officinalis*) (leaf) is a medicinal plant that has long been used in European and other Traditional Medicines, particularly for its memory-enhancing properties. Some of the actions and uses of Lemon Balm include improving memory[395,396] and cognition,[396,397] improving mood,[395-397] and has anti-anxiety effects,[346,395,396] acetylcholinesterase inhibition effects,[396] and stimulates the acetylcholine and gamma-aminobutyric acid (GABA) agonist receptors.[396]

Lemon Balm also has calming,[395,397,398] as a tonic,[332] antioxidant,[332] antispasmodic,[332] digestive,[332] carminative,[332] sedative,[332,395,398] and analgesic[332] effects and is used as an aid for inducing sleep.[376,395]

Milk Thistle

Milk Thistle (*Silybum marianum*) (fruit), sometimes referred to as St Mary's Thistle, is one of my favourite liver and digestion herbs that I have been prescribing to patients for over 26 years. Milk Thistle has been utilised since ancient times by physicians and herbalists to treat various liver dysfunctions and gallbladder disorders.[34,36,399] The earliest mentions of this Milk Thistle can be traced back to the Old Testament (Genesis 3:18). In ancient Greece, Milk Thistle was used as a remedy for liver dysfunction. Furthermore, traditional Indian and Chinese medicinal practices incorporated the use of Milk Thistle to treat liver and gallbladder issues.[36] Milk Thistle has hepatoprotective,[34-36] antioxidant,[34-36,399-401] anti-inflammatory,[34-36,400] antifibrotic[34,400,401] effects, along with potential cardioprotective and hypoglycaemic effects.[35] Some of the uses and clinical applications for Milk Thistle include liver conditions,[34,35,399-401] gallbladder conditions,[34,399] and digestive issues.[35]

Okra

Okra (*Hibiscus esculentus*/*Abelmoschus esculentus*), also known as Ladies Finger, is a medicinal plant with multiple health benefits described in Ayurveda.[345] Okra pods (fruits) possess a mucilaginous texture[345,402] and are abundant in minerals, carbohydrates,[345,402] dietary fibre,[345,402,403] polysaccharides (hemicellulose, cellulose, gum and pectin),[404] and unsaturated fatty acids, notably linolenic acid and oleic acid.[345]

In traditional medicine, Okra is utilised for the treatment of microbial infections, elevated blood glucose levels, constipation, hyperlipidaemia, and inflammation.[345] An infusion (think of herbal tea) made from the mucilage of the fruit was used to treat dysentery and diarrhoea during episodes of acute inflammation and irritation of the stomach and intestines, as well as for dysuria (painful, burning, or uncomfortable urination).[402] Okra has antioxidant,[405] free radical scavenging,[404] anti-inflammatory,[405] immunomodulatory,[405] gastroprotective,[405] neuroprotective,[404,405] and lipid lowering properties.[405] In traditional medicine, Okra is utilised for the treatment of microbial infections, constipation, and inflammation.[345]

Passionflower

Passionflower is one of my most favourite herbs. I have been prescribing Passionflower to patients for over 26 years. Passionflower (*Passiflora incarnata*) (herb; herb flowering and fruiting) has long been used in traditional herbal medicine in Europe for the treatment of insomnia and anxiety.[406] Some of the phytochemicals found in the passionflower are the flavonoids apigenin, luteolin, quercetin, and kaempferol.[407]

Passionflower has numerous therapeutic actions, with some of these including anxiolytic,[346,376,407-410] analgesic,[406] anti-spasmodic,[406,407] and sedative[406,408,411] actions. Passionflower is used to reduce anxiety,[346,376,407,409-411] depression,[407] stress,[407] nervousness,[411] irritability,[411] insomnia,[376,406,407,411] neuralgia,[406,411] dysmenorrhoea,[406] and symptoms of menopause.[411]

Rhodiola

Rhodiola (*Rhodiola rosea*) (root) is another one of my favourite herbs and been prescribing it to patients for over 20 years. Rhodiola has been used for centuries to increase physical endurance,[25] work productivity,[25] and resistance to high-altitude sickness,[25] and to treat fatigue,[25] depression,[25] anaemia,[25] for gastrointestinal ailments,[25] and nervous system disorders.,[25] Rhodiola has also be used to increase longevity.[25] Rhodiola is an adaptogen[25,358] with anti-stress, antidepressant,[412-414] anti-inflammatory,[415] and antioxidant properties.[415]

Some of the uses of Rhodiola include reducing anxiety[25,346,412] and depression,[25,410,412-415] improving mental performance,[416] increasing concentration,[416] fatigue,[25,412,413,415,416] exhaustion,[25] and stress.[414] Rhodiola has also been found to enhance work performance,[25,413] endurance,[25] resilience,[25] improve burnout-related symptoms,[25] and has neuroprotective[412,415] and cardioprotective effects.[25,412,415]

A randomised, double-blind, placebo-controlled, parallel-group study demonstrated that Rhodiola (576 mg per day) had an anti-fatigue effect, enhancing mental performance, especially concentration abilities, while also reducing cortisol responses to stress upon awakening in patients with burnout and fatigue syndrome.[416]

A randomised, double-blind, placebo-controlled study with parallel groups conducted over a period of 6 weeks investigated the effects of Rhodiola on patients experiencing mild to moderate depression.[417] Participants were assigned to one of three groups: the first group received two tablets daily of Rhodiola (340 mg/day), the second group was administered two tablets twice daily of Rhodiola (680 mg/day), and the third group was given two placebo tablets daily. The groups that received Rhodiola at doses of 340 mg and 680 mg daily showed significant improvements in overall depression, insomnia, emotional instability, and somatisation.[417] Somatisation refers to the tendency to manifest emotional or psychological suffering via physical symptoms.

Saffron

Saffron (*Crocus sativus*) (stigma) has been used in traditional medicine for thousands of years[408] and has recently gained popularity due to its numerous benefits during stressful times. I have been prescribing Saffron for decades. Saffron has been found to be beneficial in the management of depression[409,410,418-425] and insomnia.[426] Saffron has antidepressant,[424] mood-enhancing,[424] anti-inflammatory,[422-424,426,427] antioxidant,[422-424,427] sleep-promoting,[425,426] learning and memory enhancing,[427] neuro-endocrine, and neuroprotective effects.[422]

The mood-enhancing properties of saffron are believed to operate through various mechanisms, including the modulation of neurotransmitter activity, the regulation of the stress response (specifically the hypothalamus-pituitary-adrenal axis), and the reduction of inflammation and oxidative stress.[424]

A randomised, double-blind, placebo-controlled trial with a parallel-group design was conducted over 28 days to examine the effects of Saffron on improving sleep.[425] The active treatment group received one tablet of 14 mg of a standardised saffron extract (which was standardised to contain over 3.5% Lepticrosalides) twice daily, while the placebo group was administered one tablet of the placebo twice daily for the same duration. The saffron group exhibited greater reductions in the Insomnia Severity Index score compared to the placebo group. Similarly, the saffron group showed more significant reductions in the Restorative Sleep Questionnaire score than the placebo group. Furthermore, improvements in sleep quality were more pronounced in the saffron group relative to the placebo group. Statistically significant enhancements were noted in the saffron group regarding the number of awakenings after sleep onset, overall sleep quality, and alertness upon waking.[425] No significant changes were observed in the placebo group.[425]

Shatavari

I first used Shatavari (*Asparagus racemosus*) (peeled root) in patients over 25 years ago and have prescribed it regularly since. Shatavari is an Ayurvedic herb that has a rich history of being used for the treatment of gastric ulcers,[428] dyspepsia,[428,429] nervous disorders,[428] inflammation,[428] and liver diseases.[428] Shatavari contains isoflavones, sapogenins, fructo-oligosaccharides, polysaccharides, shatavarins, asparosides, racemosols, glycosides, mucilage, fatty acids,[430] and saponins.[430,431] Shatavari contains phytoestrogenic compounds that bind to the oestradiol receptor.[432]

Shatavari is used for hormone regulation,[430] fertility promotion,[430] stress management,[430] liver conditions,[358] and nervous disorders.[358] Shatavari has adaptogenic[358] tonic,[358] rejuvenating,[358] antidepressant,[358] immunomodulatory,[358] antioxidant,[358] and anti-inflammatory,[358] actions. Research indicates that Shatavari may increase skeletal muscle strength.[433] In a randomised double-blind, placebo-controlled study, 20 postmenopausal women (average age 68.5 ± 6 years) were administered either a placebo (n = 10) or Shatavari (n = 10; 1000 mg/day, which corresponds to 26,500 mg/day of fresh weight Shatavari) over a period of 6 weeks.[432] Results indicated an enhancement in handgrip strength and an increase in myosin regulatory light chain phosphorylation (a recognised indicator of improved myosin contractile function) in the Vastus lateralis following the supplementation of Shatavari.[432]

Turmeric

Where would we be without turmeric? Turmeric (*Curcuma longa*) (rhizome) is a favourite of mine and other health professionals for its numerous actions and clinical applications. Turmeric has a long history of use for skin diseases, infection, stress, and depression.[434] Turmeric has been used in Ayurvedic medicine for aches, pains, wounds, sprains, and liver disorders.[24] It has anti-inflammatory,[341,342,371,434-441] antioxidant,[341,342,434-441] immunomodulatory,[371,437] hepatoprotective,[435,440,441] neuroprotective,[440] antimicrobial,[341,342,440,441] memory enhancing,[341] anti-depressant,[341] and wound healing[341,342] properties.

Turmeric is used for inflammation,[341,342,371,434-441] oxidative stress,[435,436,438] cardiovascular disease,[341,434,441] cardiometabolic disease,[341] hyperlipidaemia,[341] gastrointestinal disorders,[441] Crohn's disease,[341] liver conditions,[341,435] depression,[341] osteoarthritis,[341] acne,[442] dermatitis,[341,442] psoriasis,[341,442] and pain.[436,437] In very rare cases, Curcuma species may harm the liver. Stop use and see a doctor if you have yellowing skin/eyes or unusual: fatigue, nausea, appetite loss, abdominal pain, dark urine, or itching.

CONCLUSION

Nicotinamide mononucleotide (NMN) is a water-soluble bioactive nucleotide that performs numerous functions in the body, including increasing NAD^+ levels, increasing cellular energy, improving mitochondrial bioenergetics and energy metabolism, acting as an anti-inflammatory and antioxidant, reducing reactive oxygen species (ROS) and oxidative stress, activating SIRT1, and improving mitochondrial dynamics and function, with potential anti-ageing effects. Numerous human clinical trials support the use of NMN for various uses, including increasing intracellular NAD^+ levels, enhancing NAD levels, enhancing muscle insulin signalling, improving muscle insulin sensitivity, reducing arterial stiffness, enhancing muscle NAD^+ turnover, decreasing postprandial hyperinsulinaemia, decreasing total cholesterol, decreasing LDL cholesterol, decreasing apolipoprotein B levels, decreasing diastolic blood pressure, improving motor function, improving walking speed, increases walking distance, enhancing aerobic capacity, potential to improve maximal voluntary muscle strength, showing potential in reducing body weight, improving sleep quality, improving longevity, and improving health-related quality of life. NMN can be taken as a single product or can be combined with various vitamins, minerals, nutrients, and herbs, based on the desired outcomes.

REFERENCES

1. Sartorius N. The meanings of health and its promotion. *Croatian medical journal* 2006; 47(4): 662-4.
2. Kouba BR, Camargo A, Gil-Mohapel J, et al. Molecular Basis Underlying the Therapeutic Potential of Vitamin D for the Treatment of Depression and Anxiety. *International journal of molecular sciences* 2022; 23(13): 7077.
3. Aggarwal BB, Sundaram C, Prasad S, et al. Tocotrienols, the vitamin E of the 21st century: its potential against cancer and other chronic diseases. *Biochem Pharmacol* 2010; 80(11): 1613-31.
4. Sen CK, Khanna S, Roy S. Tocotrienols: Vitamin E beyond tocopherols. *Life sciences* 2006; 78(18): 2088-98.
5. Ahsan H, Ahad A, Iqbal J, et al. Pharmacological potential of tocotrienols: a review. *Nutr Metab (Lond)* 2014; 11(1): 52.
6. Chin KY, Pang KL, Soelaiman IN. Tocotrienol and Its Role in Chronic Diseases. *Adv Exp Med Biol* 2016; 928: 97-130.
7. Comitato R, Ambra R, Virgili F. Tocotrienols: A Family of Molecules with Specific Biological Activities. *Antioxidants (Basel, Switzerland)* 2017; 6(4): 93.
8. Kennedy DO. B Vitamins and the Brain: Mechanisms, Dose and Efficacy--A Review. *Nutrients* 2016; 8(2): 68.
9. Powers HJ. Riboflavin (vitamin B-2) and health. *Am J Clin Nutr* 2003; 77(6): 1352-60.
10. Ashoori M, Saedisomeolia A. Riboflavin (vitamin B(2)) and oxidative stress: a review. *Br J Nutr* 2014; 111(11): 1985-91.
11. van Summeren MJ, Braam LA, Lilien MR, et al. The effect of menaquinone-7 (vitamin K2) supplementation on osteocalcin carboxylation in healthy prepubertal children. *Br J Nutr* 2009; 102(8): 1171-8.
12. Inaba N, Sato T, Yamashita T. Low-Dose Daily Intake of Vitamin K(2) (Menaquinone-7) Improves Osteocalcin γ-Carboxylation: A Double-Blind, Randomized Controlled Trials. *J Nutr Sci Vitaminol (Tokyo)* 2015; 61(6): 471-80.
13. Popescu A, German M. Vitamin K2 Holds Promise for Alzheimer's Prevention and Treatment. *Nutrients* 2021; 13(7).
14. Palmery M, Saraceno A, Vaiarelli A, et al. Oral contraceptives and changes in nutritional requirements. *Eur Rev Med Pharmacol Sci* 2013; 17(13): 1804-13.
15. Almohanna HM, Ahmed AA, Tsatalis JP, et al. The Role of Vitamins and Minerals in Hair Loss: A Review. *Dermatology and Therapy* 2019; 9(1): 51-70.
16. Gasperi V, Sibilano M, Savini I, et al. Niacin in the Central Nervous System: An Update of Biological Aspects and Clinical Applications. *International journal of molecular sciences* 2019; 20(4): 974.
17. Moskowitz A, Donnino MW. Thiamine (vitamin B1) in septic shock: a targeted therapy. *J Thorac Dis* 2020; 12(Suppl 1): S78-S83.
18. Manzetti S, Zhang J, van der Spoel D. Thiamin function, metabolism, uptake, and transport. *Biochemistry* 2014; 53(5): 821-35.
19. Wang ZQ, Cefalu WT. Current concepts about chromium supplementation in type 2 diabetes and insulin resistance. *Curr Diab Rep* 2010; 10(2): 145-51.
20. Anderson RA. Effects of chromium on body composition and weight loss. *Nutrition reviews* 1998; 56(9): 266-70.
21. Alajil O, Sagar VR, Kaur C, et al. Nutritional and Phytochemical Traits of Apricots (Prunus Armeniaca L.) for Application in Nutraceutical and Health Industry. *Foods* 2021; 10(6).
22. McEwen BJ. Comment on "Investigation of Possible Herb-Drug Interactions for the Treatment of Cardiovascular Diseases". *Semin Thromb Hemost* 2019; 45(5): 552-3.
23. Hartmann G, McEwen B. The potential of herbal medicine in the management of endometriosis. *Journal of the Australian Traditional-Medicine Society* 2018; 24(3): 146-54.
24. McEwen BJ. The influence of herbal medicine on platelet function and coagulation: a narrative review. *Semin Thromb Hemost* 2015; 41(3): 300-14.

25. Ivanova Stojcheva E, Quintela JC. The Effectiveness of Rhodiola rosea L. Preparations in Alleviating Various Aspects of Life-Stress Symptoms and Stress-Induced Conditions-Encouraging Clinical Evidence. *Molecules* 2022; 27(12).
26. Salve J, Pate S, Debnath K, et al. Adaptogenic and Anxiolytic Effects of Ashwagandha Root Extract in Healthy Adults: A Double-blind, Randomized, Placebo-controlled Clinical Study. *Cureus* 2019; 11(12): e6466.
27. Saleem S, Muhammad G, Hussain MA, et al. Withania somnifera L.: Insights into the phytochemical profile, therapeutic potential, clinical trials, and future prospective. *Iran J Basic Med Sci* 2020; 23(12): 1501-26.
28. Mikulska P, Malinowska M, Ignacyk M, et al. Ashwagandha (Withania somnifera)-Current Research on the Health-Promoting Activities: A Narrative Review. *Pharmaceutics* 2023; 15(4).
29. Speers AB, Cabey KA, Soumyanath A, et al. Effects of Withania somnifera (Ashwagandha) on Stress and the Stress- Related Neuropsychiatric Disorders Anxiety, Depression, and Insomnia. *Current neuropharmacology* 2021; 19(9): 1468-95.
30. Ziegenfuss TN, Kedia AW, Sandrock JE, et al. Effects of an Aqueous Extract of Withania somnifera on Strength Training Adaptations and Recovery: The STAR Trial. *Nutrients* 2018; 10(11).
31. McKay DL, Blumberg JB. A review of the bioactivity and potential health benefits of chamomile tea (Matricaria recutita L.). *Phytother Res* 2006; 20(7): 519-30.
32. Khalesi ZB, Beiranvand SP, Bokaie M. Efficacy of Chamomile in the Treatment of Premenstrual Syndrome: A Systematic Review. *J Pharmacopuncture* 2019; 22(4): 204-9.
33. Amsterdam JD, Li Y, Soeller I, et al. A randomized, double-blind, placebo-controlled trial of oral Matricaria recutita (chamomile) extract therapy for generalized anxiety disorder. *J Clin Psychopharmacol* 2009; 29(4): 378-82.
34. Jiang G, Sun C, Wang X, et al. Hepatoprotective mechanism of Silybum marianum on nonalcoholic fatty liver disease based on network pharmacology and experimental verification. *Bioengineered* 2022; 13(3): 5216-35.
35. Wadhwa K, Pahwa R, Kumar M, et al. Mechanistic Insights into the Pharmacological Significance of Silymarin. *Molecules* 2022; 27(16).
36. Bijak M. Silybin, a Major Bioactive Component of Milk Thistle (Silybum marianum L. Gaernt.)-Chemistry, Bioavailability, and Metabolism. *Molecules* 2017; 22(11).
37. Aguiar S, Borowski T. Neuropharmacological review of the nootropic herb Bacopa monnieri. *Rejuvenation Res* 2013; 16(4): 313-26.
38. Fatima U, Roy S, Ahmad S, et al. Pharmacological attributes of Bacopa monnieri extract: Current updates and clinical manifestation. *Front Nutr* 2022; 9: 972379.
39. Yamane T, Imai M, Bamba T, et al. Nicotinamide mononucleotide (NMN) intake increases plasma NMN and insulin levels in healthy subjects. *Clinical nutrition ESPEN* 2023; 56: 83-6.
40. Zhang R, Chen S, Wang Z, et al. Assessing the Effects of Nicotinamide Mononucleotide Supplementation on Pulmonary Inflammation in Male Mice Subchronically Exposed to Ambient Particulate Matter. *Environ Health Perspect* 2023; 131(7): 77006.
41. Ahmed M, Riaz U, Lv H, et al. Nicotinamide Mononucleotide Restores NAD(+) Levels to Alleviate LPS-Induced Inflammation via the TLR4/NF-κB/MAPK Signaling Pathway in Mice Granulosa Cells. *Antioxidants (Basel)* 2024; 14(1).
42. Li HR, Liu Q, Zhu CL, et al. β-Nicotinamide mononucleotide activates NAD+/SIRT1 pathway and attenuates inflammatory and oxidative responses in the hippocampus regions of septic mice. *Redox Biol* 2023; 63: 102745.
43. Wang X, Hu X, Yang Y, et al. Nicotinamide mononucleotide protects against β-amyloid oligomer-induced cognitive impairment and neuronal death. *Brain Res* 2016; 1643: 1-9.
44. Long AN, Owens K, Schlappal AE, et al. Effect of nicotinamide mononucleotide on brain mitochondrial respiratory deficits in an Alzheimer's disease-relevant murine model. *BMC Neurol* 2015; 15: 19.
45. Yamamoto T, Byun J, Zhai P, et al. Nicotinamide mononucleotide, an intermediate of NAD+ synthesis, protects the heart from ischemia and reperfusion. *PLoS One* 2014; 9(6): e98972.
46. Mills KF, Yoshida S, Stein LR, et al. Long-Term Administration of Nicotinamide Mononucleotide Mitigates Age-Associated Physiological Decline in Mice. *Cell Metab* 2016; 24(6): 795-806.

47. Poddar SK, Sifat AE, Haque S, et al. Nicotinamide Mononucleotide: Exploration of Diverse Therapeutic Applications of a Potential Molecule. *Biomolecules* 2019; 9(1).
48. Cros C, Margier M, Cannelle H, et al. Nicotinamide Mononucleotide Administration Triggers Macrophages Reprogramming and Alleviates Inflammation During Sepsis Induced by Experimental Peritonitis. *Front Mol Biosci* 2022; 9: 895028.
49. Wang L, Chen Y, Wei J, et al. Administration of nicotinamide mononucleotide improves oocyte quality of obese mice. *Cell Prolif* 2022; 55(11): e13303.
50. de Picciotto NE, Gano LB, Johnson LC, et al. Nicotinamide mononucleotide supplementation reverses vascular dysfunction and oxidative stress with aging in mice. *Aging Cell* 2016; 15(3): 522-30.
51. World Health Organization. Positioning Health in the Post-2015 Development Agenda: WHO discussion paper, 2012.
52. World Health Organization. Constitution of WHO: principles. 2017. http://www.who.int/about/mission/en/.
53. Marmot M, Allen JJ. Social determinants of health equity. *American journal of public health* 2014; 104 Suppl 4: S517-9.
54. Billman GE. Homeostasis: The Underappreciated and Far Too Often Ignored Central Organizing Principle of Physiology. *Frontiers in physiology* 2020; 11: 200.
55. The Lancet. What is health? The ability to adapt. *The Lancet* 2009; 373(9666): 781.
56. World Health Organization. The Ottawa Charter for Health Promotion. 2016. http://www.who.int/healthpromotion/conferences/previous/ottawa/en/ (accessed 25/05/2016.
57. Wang W, Yan Y, Guo Z, et al. All around suboptimal health - a joint position paper of the Suboptimal Health Study Consortium and European Association for Predictive, Preventive and Personalised Medicine. *Epma j* 2021; 12(4): 403-33.
58. Keyes D, Patel NI, Correa KA. Overview of Lifestyle Medicine. StatPearls. Treasure Island (FL): StatPearls Publishing
Copyright © 2025, StatPearls Publishing LLC.; 2025.
59. Bruins MJ, Van Dael P, Eggersdorfer M. The Role of Nutrients in Reducing the Risk for Noncommunicable Diseases during Aging. *Nutrients* 2019; 11(1): 85.
60. Garmany A, Yamada S, Terzic A. Longevity leap: mind the healthspan gap. *NPJ Regen Med* 2021; 6(1): 57.
61. Olshansky SJ. From Lifespan to Healthspan. *Jama* 2018; 320(13): 1323-4.
62. Rajado AT, Silva N, Esteves F, et al. How can we modulate aging through nutrition and physical exercise? An epigenetic approach. *Aging (Albany NY)* 2023; 15(8): 3191-217.
63. Cockerham WC, Hamby BW, Oates GR. The Social Determinants of Chronic Disease. *American journal of preventive medicine* 2017; 52(1S1): S5-S12.
64. Li X, Ploner A, Wang Y, et al. Clinical biomarkers and associations with healthspan and lifespan: Evidence from observational and genetic data. *EBioMedicine* 2021; 66: 103318.
65. Hansen M, Kennedy BK. Does Longer Lifespan Mean Longer Healthspan? *Trends Cell Biol* 2016; 26(8): 565-8.
66. Blagosklonny MV. No limit to maximal lifespan in humans: how to beat a 122-year-old record. *Oncoscience* 2021; 8: 110-9.
67. Kaeberlein M. How healthy is the healthspan concept? *Geroscience* 2018; 40(4): 361-4.
68. Papadopoulou SK, Mantzorou M, Voulgaridou G, et al. Nutritional Status Is Associated with Health-Related Quality of Life, Physical Activity, and Sleep Quality: A Cross-Sectional Study in an Elderly Greek Population. *Nutrients* 2023; 15(2).
69. Jafari M. Healthspan Pharmacology. *Rejuvenation Res* 2015; 18(6): 573-80.
70. Teskey G, Abrahem R, Cao R, et al. Chapter Five - Glutathione as a Marker for Human Disease. In: Makowski GS, ed. Advances in Clinical Chemistry: Elsevier; 2018: 141-59.
71. Rahman SU, Qadeer A, Wu Z. Role and Potential Mechanisms of Nicotinamide Mononucleotide in Aging. *Aging Dis* 2024; 15(2): 565-83.
72. Houtkooper RH, Auwerx J. Exploring the therapeutic space around NAD+. *J Cell Biol* 2012; 199(2): 205-9.
73. López-Otín C, Blasco MA, Partridge L, et al. Hallmarks of aging: An expanding universe. *Cell* 2023; 186(2): 243-78.

74. Nunnari J, Suomalainen A. Mitochondria: in sickness and in health. *Cell* 2012; 148(6): 1145-59.
75. Harrington JS, Ryter SW, Plataki M, et al. Mitochondria in health, disease, and aging. *Physiol Rev* 2023; 103(4): 2349-422.
76. Annesley SJ, Fisher PR. Mitochondria in Health and Disease. *Cells* 2019; 8(7).
77. Webb M, Sideris DP. Intimate Relations-Mitochondria and Ageing. *International journal of molecular sciences* 2020; 21(20).
78. Singh A, D'Amico D, Andreux PA, et al. Urolithin A improves muscle strength, exercise performance, and biomarkers of mitochondrial health in a randomized trial in middle-aged adults. *Cell Rep Med* 2022; 3(5): 100633.
79. Miwa S, Kashyap S, Chini E, et al. Mitochondrial dysfunction in cell senescence and aging. *J Clin Invest* 2022; 132(13).
80. Lucius K. Botanical Medicine and Phytochemicals in Healthy Aging and Longevity—Part 1. *Alternative and Complementary Therapies* 2020; 26(1): 31-7.
81. Chan SR, Blackburn EH. Telomeres and telomerase. *Philos Trans R Soc Lond B Biol Sci* 2004; 359(1441): 109-21.
82. Blackburn EH. Telomeres. *Trends Biochem Sci* 1991; 16(10): 378-81.
83. Rhodes D, Fairall L, Simonsson T, et al. Telomere architecture. *EMBO Rep* 2002; 3(12): 1139-45.
84. Lin JJ. Telomeric DNA binding proteins. *Bioessays* 1993; 15(8): 555-7.
85. Engin AB, Engin A. The Connection Between Cell Fate and Telomere. *Adv Exp Med Biol* 2021; 1275: 71-100.
86. Epel ES, Blackburn EH, Lin J, et al. Accelerated telomere shortening in response to life stress. *Proc Natl Acad Sci U S A* 2004; 101(49): 17312-5.
87. Kiecolt-Glaser JK, Epel ES, Belury MA, et al. Omega-3 fatty acids, oxidative stress, and leukocyte telomere length: A randomized controlled trial. *Brain, behavior, and immunity* 2013; 28: 16-24.
88. Blackburn EH, Epel ES, Lin J. Human telomere biology: A contributory and interactive factor in aging, disease risks, and protection. *Science* 2015; 350(6265): 1193-8.
89. Kunnumakkara AB, Sailo BL, Banik K, et al. Chronic diseases, inflammation, and spices: how are they linked? *J Transl Med* 2018; 16(1): 14.
90. Chen L, Deng H, Cui H, et al. Inflammatory responses and inflammation-associated diseases in organs. *Oncotarget* 2018; 9(6): 7204-18.
91. Pervez MA, Khan DA, Ijaz A, et al. Effects of Delta-tocotrienol Supplementation on Liver Enzymes, Inflammation, Oxidative stress and Hepatic Steatosis in Patients with Nonalcoholic Fatty Liver Disease. *Turk J Gastroenterol* 2018; 29(2): 170-6.
92. Liguori I, Russo G, Curcio F, et al. Oxidative stress, aging, and diseases. *Clin Interv Aging* 2018; 13: 757-72.
93. Zhu XH, Lu M, Lee BY, et al. In vivo NAD assay reveals the intracellular NAD contents and redox state in healthy human brain and their age dependences. *Proc Natl Acad Sci U S A* 2015; 112(9): 2876-81.
94. McReynolds MR, Chellappa K, Baur JA. Age-related NAD(+) decline. *Exp Gerontol* 2020; 134: 110888.
95. Rajman L, Chwalek K, Sinclair DA. Therapeutic Potential of NAD-Boosting Molecules: The In Vivo Evidence. *Cell Metab* 2018; 27(3): 529-47.
96. Soma M, Lalam SK. The role of nicotinamide mononucleotide (NMN) in anti-aging, longevity, and its potential for treating chronic conditions. *Mol Biol Rep* 2022; 49(10): 9737-48.
97. Wu LE, Sinclair DA. The elusive NMN transporter is found. *Nature Metabolism* 2019; 1(1): 8-9.
98. Hong W, Mo F, Zhang Z, et al. Nicotinamide Mononucleotide: A Promising Molecule for Therapy of Diverse Diseases by Targeting NAD+ Metabolism. *Front Cell Dev Biol* 2020; 8: 246.
99. Lin SJ, Guarente L. Nicotinamide adenine dinucleotide, a metabolic regulator of transcription, longevity and disease. *Curr Opin Cell Biol* 2003; 15(2): 241-6.
100. Abdellatif M, Sedej S, Kroemer G. NAD+ Metabolism in Cardiac Health, Aging, and Disease. *Circulation* 2021; 144(22): 1795-817.

References

101. Yamaguchi S, Irie J, Mitsuishi M, et al. Safety and efficacy of long-term nicotinamide mononucleotide supplementation on metabolism, sleep, and nicotinamide adenine dinucleotide biosynthesis in healthy, middle-aged Japanese men. *Endocr J* 2024; 71(2): 153-69.
102. Grozio A, Mills KF, Yoshino J, et al. Slc12a8 is a nicotinamide mononucleotide transporter. *Nat Metab* 2019; 1(1): 47-57.
103. National Center for Biotechnology Information. PubChem Compound Summary for CID 936, Nicotinamide. 2025. https://pubchem.ncbi.nlm.nih.gov/compound/Nicotinamide.
104. National Center for Biotechnology Information. PubChem Compound Summary for CID 439924, Nicotinamide Riboside. 2025. https://pubchem.ncbi.nlm.nih.gov/compound/Nicotinamide-Riboside.
105. National Center for Biotechnology Information. PubChem Compound Summary for CID 14180, Nicotinamide Mononucleotide. 2025. https://pubchem.ncbi.nlm.nih.gov/compound/Nicotinamide-Mononucleotide.
106. National Center for Biotechnology Information. PubChem Compound Summary for CID 170855691, Nicotinamide-Adenine-Dinucleotide. 2025. https://pubchem.ncbi.nlm.nih.gov/compound/Nicotinamide-Adenine-Dinucleotide.
107. Liao G, Xie Y, Peng H, et al. Advancements in NMN biotherapy and research updates in the field of digestive system diseases. *Journal of Translational Medicine* 2024; 22(1): 805.
108. Kuerec AH, Wang W, Yi L, et al. Towards personalized nicotinamide mononucleotide (NMN) supplementation: Nicotinamide adenine dinucleotide (NAD) concentration. *Mechanisms of Ageing and Development* 2024; 218: 111917.
109. Morifuji M, Higashi S, Ebihara S, et al. Ingestion of β-nicotinamide mononucleotide increased blood NAD levels, maintained walking speed, and improved sleep quality in older adults in a double-blind randomized, placebo-controlled study. *Geroscience* 2024; 46(5): 4671-88.
110. Yoshino M, Yoshino J, Kayser BD, et al. Nicotinamide mononucleotide increases muscle insulin sensitivity in prediabetic women. *Science* 2021; 372(6547): 1224-9.
111. Yi L, Maier AB, Tao R, et al. The efficacy and safety of β-nicotinamide mononucleotide (NMN) supplementation in healthy middle-aged adults: a randomized, multicenter, double-blind, placebo-controlled, parallel-group, dose-dependent clinical trial. *Geroscience* 2023; 45(1): 29-43.
112. Pencina KM, Valderrabano R, Wipper B, et al. Nicotinamide Adenine Dinucleotide Augmentation in Overweight or Obese Middle-Aged and Older Adults: A Physiologic Study. *J Clin Endocrinol Metab* 2023; 108(8): 1968-80.
113. Pencina KM, Lavu S, Dos Santos M, et al. MIB-626, an Oral Formulation of a Microcrystalline Unique Polymorph of β-Nicotinamide Mononucleotide, Increases Circulating Nicotinamide Adenine Dinucleotide and its Metabolome in Middle-Aged and Older Adults. *J Gerontol A Biol Sci Med Sci* 2023; 78(1): 90-6.
114. Katayoshi T, Uehata S, Nakashima N, et al. Nicotinamide adenine dinucleotide metabolism and arterial stiffness after long-term nicotinamide mononucleotide supplementation: a randomized, double-blind, placebo-controlled trial. *Scientific reports* 2023; 13(1): 2786.
115. Igarashi M, Nakagawa-Nagahama Y, Miura M, et al. Chronic nicotinamide mononucleotide supplementation elevates blood nicotinamide adenine dinucleotide levels and alters muscle function in healthy older men. *NPJ Aging* 2022; 8(1): 5.
116. Liao B, Zhao Y, Wang D, et al. Nicotinamide mononucleotide supplementation enhances aerobic capacity in amateur runners: a randomized, double-blind study. *J Int Soc Sports Nutr* 2021; 18(1): 54.
117. Gao Y, Moten A, Lin H-K. Akt: a new activation mechanism. *Cell Research* 2014; 24(7): 785-6.
118. Lins L, Carvalho FM. SF-36 total score as a single measure of health-related quality of life: Scoping review. *SAGE Open Med* 2016; 4: 2050312116671725.
119. Irie J, Inagaki E, Fujita M, et al. Effect of oral administration of nicotinamide mononucleotide on clinical parameters and nicotinamide metabolite levels in healthy Japanese men. *Endocr J* 2020; 67(2): 153-60.
120. Fukamizu Y, Uchida Y, Shigekawa A, et al. Safety evaluation of β-nicotinamide mononucleotide oral administration in healthy adult men and women. *Scientific reports* 2022; 12(1): 14442.

121. Fairfield KM, Fletcher RH. Vitamins for chronic disease prevention in adults: scientific review. *JAMA* 2002; 287(23): 3116-26.
122. Ciosek Ż, Kot K, Kosik-Bogacka D, et al. The Effects of Calcium, Magnesium, Phosphorus, Fluoride, and Lead on Bone Tissue. *Biomolecules* 2021; 11(4).
123. Wasilewski GB, Vervloet MG, Schurgers LJ. The Bone-Vasculature Axis: Calcium Supplementation and the Role of Vitamin K. *Frontiers in cardiovascular medicine* 2019; 6: 6.
124. Australian Government Department of Health. Nutrient Reference Values for Australia and New Zealand Including Recommended Dietary Intakes. 1.2 ed; 2006.
125. Davis RE, Icke GC. Clinical chemistry of thiamin. *Adv Clin Chem* 1983; 23: 93-140.
126. Manna P, Kalita J. Beneficial role of vitamin K supplementation on insulin sensitivity, glucose metabolism, and the reduced risk of type 2 diabetes: A review. *Nutrition* 2016; 32(7-8): 732-9.
127. Schwalfenberg GK. Vitamins K1 and K2: The Emerging Group of Vitamins Required for Human Health. *J Nutr Metab* 2017; 2017: 6254836.
128. Brugè F, Bacchetti T, Principi F, et al. Olive oil supplemented with menaquinone-7 significantly affects osteocalcin carboxylation. *Br J Nutr* 2011; 106(7): 1058-62.
129. Zimmermann MB. Iodine deficiency. *Endocr Rev* 2009; 30(4): 376-408.
130. Jugdaohsingh R. Silicon and bone health. *The journal of nutrition, health & aging* 2007; 11(2): 99-110.
131. Michalak M, Pierzak M, Kręcisz B, et al. Bioactive Compounds for Skin Health: A Review. *Nutrients* 2021; 13(1): 203.
132. Khammissa RAG, Fourie J, Motswaledi MH, et al. The Biological Activities of Vitamin D and Its Receptor in Relation to Calcium and Bone Homeostasis, Cancer, Immune and Cardiovascular Systems, Skin Biology, and Oral Health. *BioMed research international* 2018; 2018: 9276380.
133. Hossein-nezhad A, Holick MF. Vitamin D for health: a global perspective. *Mayo Clin Proc* 2013; 88(7): 720-55.
134. McArthur JO, Tang H, Petocz P, et al. Biological variability and impact of oral contraceptives on vitamins B(6), B(12) and folate status in women of reproductive age. *Nutrients* 2013; 5(9): 3634-45.
135. Judd SE, Tangpricha V. Vitamin D deficiency and risk for cardiovascular disease. *Am J Med Sci* 2009; 338(1): 40-4.
136. Xue W, You J, Su Y, et al. The Effect of Magnesium Deficiency on Neurological Disorders: A Narrative Review Article. *Iranian journal of public health* 2019; 48(3): 379-87.
137. Berkelhammer C, Bear RA. A clinical approach to common electrolyte problems: 4. Hypomagnesemia. *Canadian Medical Association journal* 1985; 132(4): 360-8.
138. Kashyap ML, Ganji S, Nakra NK, et al. Niacin for treatment of nonalcoholic fatty liver disease (NAFLD): novel use for an old drug? *Journal of clinical lipidology* 2019; 13(6): 873-9.
139. Wan L, Li Y, Zhang Z, et al. Methylenetetrahydrofolate reductase and psychiatric diseases. *Transl Psychiatry* 2018; 8(1): 242.
140. Obeid R, Holzgreve W, Pietrzik K. Is 5-methyltetrahydrofolate an alternative to folic acid for the prevention of neural tube defects? *J Perinat Med* 2013; 41(5): 469-83.
141. Volpe SL. Magnesium in disease prevention and overall health. *Adv Nutr* 2013; 4(3): 378s-83s.
142. Enders M, Heider T, Ludwig A, et al. Strategies for Neuroprotection in Multiple Sclerosis and the Role of Calcium. *International journal of molecular sciences* 2020; 21(5).
143. Schwalfenberg GK, Genuis SJ. The Importance of Magnesium in Clinical Healthcare. *Scientifica* 2017; 2017: 4179326-.
144. Khezri MB, Nasseh N, Soltanian G. The comparative preemptive analgesic efficacy of addition of vitamin B complex to gabapentin versus gabapentin alone in women undergoing cesarean section under spinal anesthesia: A prospective randomized double-blind study. *Medicine* 2017; 96(15): e6545.
145. Holick MF. Vitamin D: a d-lightful solution for health. *J Investig Med* 2011; 59(6): 872-80.
146. Ueland PM, Ulvik A, Rios-Avila L, et al. Direct and Functional Biomarkers of Vitamin B6 Status. *Annu Rev Nutr* 2015; 35: 33-70.

147. Bourre JM. Effects of nutrients (in food) on the structure and function of the nervous system: update on dietary requirements for brain. Part 1: micronutrients. *The journal of nutrition, health & aging* 2006; 10(5): 377-85.
148. Kobla HV, Volpe SL. Chromium, exercise, and body composition. *Crit Rev Food Sci Nutr* 2000; 40(4): 291-308.
149. Bromage S, Ahmed T, Fawzi WW. Calcium Deficiency in Bangladesh: Burden and Proposed Solutions for the First 1000 Days. *Food Nutr Bull* 2016; 37(4): 475-93.
150. Kumar P, Kumar M, Bedi O, et al. Role of vitamins and minerals as immunity boosters in COVID-19. *Inflammopharmacology* 2021; 29(4): 1001-16.
151. Kvícala J, Zamrazil V. Effect of iodine and selenium upon thyroid function. *Central European journal of public health* 2003; 11(2): 107-13.
152. Rohner F, Zimmermann M, Jooste P, et al. Biomarkers of nutrition for development--iodine review. *The Journal of nutrition* 2014; 144(8): 1322S-42S.
153. Niwattisaiwong S, Burman KD, Li-Ng M. Iodine deficiency: Clinical implications. *Cleveland Clinic journal of medicine* 2017; 84(3): 236-44.
154. Sorrenti S, Baldini E, Pironi D, et al. Iodine: Its Role in Thyroid Hormone Biosynthesis and Beyond. *Nutrients* 2021; 13(12).
155. Bolander FF. Vitamins: not just for enzymes. *Current opinion in investigational drugs (London, England : 2000)* 2006; 7(10): 912-5.
156. Polegato BF, Pereira AG, Azevedo PS, et al. Role of Thiamin in Health and Disease. *Nutr Clin Pract* 2019; 34(4): 558-64.
157. Frank LL. Thiamin in Clinical Practice. *JPEN Journal of parenteral and enteral nutrition* 2015; 39(5): 503-20.
158. Naghashpour M, Jafarirad S, Amani R, et al. Update on riboflavin and multiple sclerosis: a systematic review. *Iran J Basic Med Sci* 2017; 20(9): 958-66.
159. D'Andrea E, Hey SP, Ramirez CL, et al. Assessment of the Role of Niacin in Managing Cardiovascular Disease Outcomes: A Systematic Review and Meta-analysis. *JAMA Netw Open* 2019; 2(4): e192224-e.
160. Thorp VJ. Effect of oral contraceptive agents on vitamin and mineral requirements. *J Am Diet Assoc* 1980; 76(6): 581-4.
161. Aspy DJ, Madden NA, Delfabbro P. Effects of Vitamin B6 (Pyridoxine) and a B Complex Preparation on Dreaming and Sleep. *Percept Mot Skills* 2018; 125(3): 451-62.
162. Wintergerst ES, Maggini S, Hornig DH. Contribution of selected vitamins and trace elements to immune function. *Ann Nutr Metab* 2007; 51(4): 301-23.
163. Crider KS, Yang TP, Berry RJ, et al. Folate and DNA methylation: a review of molecular mechanisms and the evidence for folate's role. *Adv Nutr* 2012; 3(1): 21-38.
164. Menezo Y, Elder K, Clement A, et al. Folic Acid, Folinic Acid, 5 Methyl TetraHydroFolate Supplementation for Mutations That Affect Epigenesis through the Folate and One-Carbon Cycles. *Biomolecules* 2022; 12(2).
165. Turck D, Bohn T, Castenmiller J, et al. Conversion of calcium-l-methylfolate and (6S)-5-methyltetrahydrofolic acid glucosamine salt into dietary folate equivalents. *EFSA journal European Food Safety Authority* 2022; 20(8): e07452.
166. Bailey LB, Stover PJ, McNulty H, et al. Biomarkers of Nutrition for Development-Folate Review. *J Nutr* 2015; 145(7): 1636S-80S.
167. Moores CJ, Fenech M, O'Callaghan NJ. Telomere dynamics: the influence of folate and DNA methylation. *Ann N Y Acad Sci* 2011; 1229: 76-88.
168. Shulpekova Y, Nechaev V, Kardasheva S, et al. The Concept of Folic Acid in Health and Disease. *Molecules* 2021; 26(12).
169. Ebara S. Nutritional role of folate. *Congenital anomalies* 2017; 57(5): 138-41.
170. Bayes J, Agrawal N, Schloss J. The Bioavailability of Various Oral Forms of Folate Supplementation in Healthy Populations and Animal Models: A Systematic Review. *J Altern Complement Med* 2019; 25(2): 169-80.
171. Briani C, Dalla Torre C, Citton V, et al. Cobalamin deficiency: clinical picture and radiological findings. *Nutrients* 2013; 5(11): 4521-39.

172. Ortega-Sáenz P, Macías D, Levitsky KL, et al. Selective accumulation of biotin in arterial chemoreceptors: requirement for carotid body exocytotic dopamine secretion. *J Physiol* 2016; 594(24): 7229-48.
173. Said HM. Biotin: biochemical, physiological and clinical aspects. *Subcell Biochem* 2012; 56: 1-19.
174. Agrawal S, Agrawal A, Said HM. Biotin deficiency enhances the inflammatory response of human dendritic cells. *Am J Physiol Cell Physiol* 2016; 311(3): C386-91.
175. Sirithanakorn C, Cronan JE. Biotin, a universal and essential cofactor: synthesis, ligation and regulation. *FEMS Microbiol Rev* 2021; 45(4).
176. Ramamoorthy K, Sabui S, Srinivasan P, et al. Effect of chronic alcohol exposure on gut vitamin B7 uptake: involvement of epigenetic mechanisms and effect of alcohol metabolites. *Am J Physiol Gastrointest Liver Physiol* 2021; 321(2): G123-g33.
177. Kuroishi T. Regulation of immunological and inflammatory functions by biotin. *Can J Physiol Pharmacol* 2015; 93(12): 1091-6.
178. Chambial S, Dwivedi S, Shukla KK, et al. Vitamin C in disease prevention and cure: an overview. *Indian journal of clinical biochemistry : IJCB* 2013; 28(4): 314-28.
179. Maggini S, Wintergerst ES, Beveridge S, et al. Selected vitamins and trace elements support immune function by strengthening epithelial barriers and cellular and humoral immune responses. *Br J Nutr* 2007; 98 Suppl 1: S29-35.
180. Gęgotek A, Skrzydlewska E. Ascorbic acid as antioxidant. *Vitam Horm* 2023; 121: 247-70.
181. Fletcher RH, Fairfield KM. Vitamins for chronic disease prevention in adults: clinical applications. *JAMA* 2002; 287(23): 3127-9.
182. Sharma B, Singh S, Siddiqi NJ. Biomedical implications of heavy metals induced imbalances in redox systems. *BioMed research international* 2014; 2014: 640754.
183. Wacker M, Holick MF. Sunlight and Vitamin D: A global perspective for health. *Dermatoendocrinol* 2013; 5(1): 51-108.
184. Holick MF. Sunlight and vitamin D for bone health and prevention of autoimmune diseases, cancers, and cardiovascular disease. *Am J Clin Nutr* 2004; 80(6 Suppl): 1678S-88S.
185. Pludowski P, Holick MF, Pilz S, et al. Vitamin D effects on musculoskeletal health, immunity, autoimmunity, cardiovascular disease, cancer, fertility, pregnancy, dementia and mortality-a review of recent evidence. *Autoimmun Rev* 2013; 12(10): 976-89.
186. Meganathan P, Fu JY. Biological Properties of Tocotrienols: Evidence in Human Studies. *International journal of molecular sciences* 2016; 17(11).
187. Sen CK, Khanna S, Rink C, et al. Tocotrienols: the emerging face of natural vitamin E. *Vitam Horm* 2007; 76: 203-61.
188. Tan BL, Norhaizan ME, Liew WP, et al. Antioxidant and Oxidative Stress: A Mutual Interplay in Age-Related Diseases. *Front Pharmacol* 2018; 9: 1162.
189. Pang KL, Chin KY. The Role of Tocotrienol in Protecting Against Metabolic Diseases. *Molecules* 2019; 24(5).
190. Suzuki YJ, Tsuchiya M, Wassall SR, et al. Structural and dynamic membrane properties of alpha-tocopherol and alpha-tocotrienol: implication to the molecular mechanism of their antioxidant potency. *Biochemistry* 1993; 32(40): 10692-9.
191. Khanna S, Roy S, Parinandi NL, et al. Characterization of the potent neuroprotective properties of the natural vitamin E alpha-tocotrienol. *J Neurochem* 2006; 98(5): 1474-86.
192. Tomeo AC, Geller M, Watkins TR, et al. Antioxidant effects of tocotrienols in patients with hyperlipidemia and carotid stenosis. *Lipids* 1995; 30(12): 1179-83.
193. Bardhan J, Chakraborty R, Raychaudhuri U. The 21st century form of vitamin E--tocotrienol. *Curr Pharm Des* 2011; 17(21): 2196-205.
194. Shahidi F, de Camargo AC. Tocopherols and Tocotrienols in Common and Emerging Dietary Sources: Occurrence, Applications, and Health Benefits. *International journal of molecular sciences* 2016; 17(10).
195. Khanna S, Roy S, Slivka A, et al. Neuroprotective properties of the natural vitamin E alpha-tocotrienol. *Stroke* 2005; 36(10): 2258-64.
196. Qureshi AA, Khan DA, Mahjabeen W, et al. Dose-dependent modulation of lipid parameters, cytokines and RNA by δ-tocotrienol in hypercholesterolemic subjects restricted to AHA Step-1 diet *Br J Med Med Res* 2015; 6(4): 351-66.

197. Malavolta M, Pierpaoli E, Giacconi R, et al. Anti-inflammatory Activity of Tocotrienols in Age-related Pathologies: A SASPected Involvement of Cellular Senescence. *Biol Proced Online* 2018; 20: 22.
198. Hariri E, Kassis N, Iskandar JP, et al. Vitamin K(2)-a neglected player in cardiovascular health: a narrative review. *Open Heart* 2021; 8(2).
199. Abdel-Rahman MS, Alkady EAM, Ahmed S. Menaquinone-7 as a novel pharmacological therapy in the treatment of rheumatoid arthritis: A clinical study. *European journal of pharmacology* 2015; 761: 273-8.
200. Beulens JW, van der AD, Grobbee DE, et al. Dietary phylloquinone and menaquinones intakes and risk of type 2 diabetes. *Diabetes Care* 2010; 33(8): 1699-705.
201. Schurgers LJ, Teunissen KJ, Hamulyak K, et al. Vitamin K-containing dietary supplements: comparison of synthetic vitamin K1 and natto-derived menaquinone-7. *Blood* 2007; 109(8): 3279-83.
202. Naiyarakseree N, Phannajit J, Naiyarakseree W, et al. Effect of Menaquinone-7 Supplementation on Arterial Stiffness in Chronic Hemodialysis Patients: A Multicenter Randomized Controlled Trial. *Nutrients* 2023; 15(11).
203. Caluwé R, Vandecasteele S, Van Vlem B, et al. Vitamin K2 supplementation in haemodialysis patients: a randomized dose-finding study. *Nephrology Dialysis Transplantation* 2014; 29(7): 1385-90.
204. Dalmeijer GW, van der Schouw YT, Magdeleyns E, et al. The effect of menaquinone-7 supplementation on circulating species of matrix Gla protein. *Atherosclerosis* 2012; 225(2): 397-402.
205. Rodríguez-Olleros Rodríguez C, Díaz Curiel M. Vitamin K and Bone Health: A Review on the Effects of Vitamin K Deficiency and Supplementation and the Effect of Non-Vitamin K Antagonist Oral Anticoagulants on Different Bone Parameters. *J Osteoporos* 2019; 2019: 2069176.
206. Rønn SH, Harsløf T, Pedersen SB, et al. Vitamin K2 (menaquinone-7) increases plasma adiponectin but does not affect insulin sensitivity in postmenopausal women: a randomized controlled trial. *Eur J Clin Nutr* 2021; 75(11): 1661-7.
207. Rønn SH, Harsløf T, Pedersen SB, et al. Vitamin K2 (menaquinone-7) prevents age-related deterioration of trabecular bone microarchitecture at the tibia in postmenopausal women. *Eur J Endocrinol* 2016; 175(6): 541-9.
208. Choi HJ, Yu J, Choi H, et al. Vitamin K2 supplementation improves insulin sensitivity via osteocalcin metabolism: a placebo-controlled trial. *Diabetes Care* 2011; 34(9): e147.
209. Vincent JB. The biochemistry of chromium. *J Nutr* 2000; 130(4): 715-8.
210. Vincent JB, Lukaski HC. Chromium. *Adv Nutr* 2018; 9(4): 505-6.
211. Jamilian M, Asemi Z. Chromium Supplementation and the Effects on Metabolic Status in Women with Polycystic Ovary Syndrome: A Randomized, Double-Blind, Placebo-Controlled Trial. *Ann Nutr Metab* 2015; 67(1): 42-8.
212. Gunalan E, Yaba A, Yilmaz B. The effect of nutrient supplementation in the management of polycystic ovary syndrome-associated metabolic dysfunctions: A critical review. *J Turk Ger Gynecol Assoc* 2018; 19(4): 220-32.
213. Hatch-McChesney A, Lieberman HR. Iodine and Iodine Deficiency: A Comprehensive Review of a Re-Emerging Issue. *Nutrients* 2022; 14(17).
214. Aakre I, Solli DD, Markhus MW, et al. Commercially available kelp and seaweed products - valuable iodine source or risk of excess intake? *Food & nutrition research* 2021; 65: 10.29219/fnr.v65.7584.
215. Ershow AG, Goodman G, Coates PM, et al. Assessing iodine intake, iodine status, and the effects of maternal iodine supplementation: introduction to articles arising from 3 workshops held by the NIH Office of Dietary Supplements. *The American journal of clinical nutrition* 2016; 104 Suppl 3(Suppl 3): 859S-63S.
216. Zimmermann MB. Iodine requirements and the risks and benefits of correcting iodine deficiency in populations. *Journal of trace elements in medicine and biology : organ of the Society for Minerals and Trace Elements (GMS)* 2008; 22(2): 81-92.
217. Schomburg L, Kohrle J. On the importance of selenium and iodine metabolism for thyroid hormone biosynthesis and human health. *Mol Nutr Food Res* 2008; 52(11): 1235-46.

218. Bilbey DL, Prabhakaran VM. Muscle cramps and magnesium deficiency: case reports. *Canadian family physician Medecin de famille canadien* 1996; 42: 1348-51.
219. Guerrera MP, Volpe SL, Mao JJ. Therapeutic uses of magnesium. *Am Fam Physician* 2009; 80(2): 157-62.
220. Grober U, Schmidt J, Kisters K. Magnesium in Prevention and Therapy. *Nutrients* 2015; 7(9): 8199-226.
221. DiNicolantonio JJ, O'Keefe JH, Wilson W. Subclinical magnesium deficiency: a principal driver of cardiovascular disease and a public health crisis. *Open Heart* 2018; 5(1).
222. Razzaque MS. Magnesium: Are We Consuming Enough? *Nutrients* 2018; 10(12).
223. de Baaij JH, Hoenderop JG, Bindels RJ. Magnesium in man: implications for health and disease. *Physiol Rev* 2015; 95(1): 1-46.
224. Harris HR, Chavarro JE, Malspeis S, et al. Dairy-food, calcium, magnesium, and vitamin D intake and endometriosis: a prospective cohort study. *American journal of epidemiology* 2013; 177(5): 420-30.
225. Balachandran RC, Mukhopadhyay S, McBride D, et al. Brain manganese and the balance between essential roles and neurotoxicity. *The Journal of biological chemistry* 2020; 295(19): 6312-29.
226. Horning KJ, Caito SW, Tipps KG, et al. Manganese Is Essential for Neuronal Health. *Annual review of nutrition* 2015; 35: 71-108.
227. Apostolova N, Victor VM. Molecular strategies for targeting antioxidants to mitochondria: therapeutic implications. *Antioxidants & redox signaling* 2015; 22(8): 686-729.
228. Li B, Huang Y, Luo C, et al. Inverse Association of Plasma Molybdenum with Metabolic Syndrome in a Chinese Adult Population: A Case-Control Study. *Nutrients* 2021; 13(12).
229. Mendel RR. The molybdenum cofactor. *The Journal of biological chemistry* 2013; 288(19): 13165-72.
230. Mendel RR, Bittner F. Cell biology of molybdenum. *Biochimica et biophysica acta* 2006; 1763(7): 621-35.
231. Vasto S, Di Gaudio F, Raso M, et al. Impact on Glucose Homeostasis: Is Food Biofortified with Molybdenum a Workable Solution? A Two-Arm Study. *Nutrients* 2022; 14(7).
232. Price CT, Koval KJ, Langford JR. Silicon: a review of its potential role in the prevention and treatment of postmenopausal osteoporosis. *International journal of endocrinology* 2013; 2013: 316783-.
233. O'Dell BL, Browning JD. Impaired calcium entry into cells is associated with pathological signs of zinc deficiency. *Adv Nutr* 2013; 4(3): 287-93.
234. Choi S, Hong DK, Choi BY, et al. Zinc in the Brain: Friend or Foe? *International journal of molecular sciences* 2020; 21(23): 8941.
235. Tuerk MJ, Fazel N. Zinc deficiency. *Curr Opin Gastroenterol* 2009; 25(2): 136-43.
236. Gammoh NZ, Rink L. Zinc in Infection and Inflammation. *Nutrients* 2017; 9(6).
237. Skrovanek S, DiGuilio K, Bailey R, et al. Zinc and gastrointestinal disease. *World J Gastrointest Pathophysiol* 2014; 5(4): 496-513.
238. Saper RB, Rash R. Zinc: an essential micronutrient. *Am Fam Physician* 2009; 79(9): 768-72.
239. Marreiro DDN, Cruz KJC, Morais JBS, et al. Zinc and Oxidative Stress: Current Mechanisms. *Antioxidants* 2017; 6(2): 24.
240. Lee SR, Noh SJ, Pronto JR, et al. The Critical Roles of Zinc: Beyond Impact on Myocardial Signaling. *The Korean journal of physiology & pharmacology : official journal of the Korean Physiological Society and the Korean Society of Pharmacology* 2015; 19(5): 389-99.
241. Jan AT, Azam M, Siddiqui K, et al. Heavy Metals and Human Health: Mechanistic Insight into Toxicity and Counter Defense System of Antioxidants. *International journal of molecular sciences* 2015; 16(12): 29592-630.
242. Prasad AS. Zinc: An antioxidant and anti-inflammatory agent: Role of zinc in degenerative disorders of aging. *Journal of Trace Elements in Medicine and Biology* 2014; 28(4): 364-71.
243. Greuter T, Franc Y, Kaelin M, et al. Low serum zinc levels predict presence of depression symptoms, but not overall disease outcome, regardless of ATG16L1 genotype in Crohn's disease patients. *Therap Adv Gastroenterol* 2018; 11: 1756283X18757715.
244. Li Z, Liu Y, Wei R, et al. The Important Role of Zinc in Neurological Diseases. *Biomolecules* 2023; 13(1): 28.

245. Russo AJ. Decreased zinc and increased copper in individuals with anxiety. *Nutr Metab Insights* 2011; 4: 1-5.
246. Nistor N, Ciontu L, Frasinariu O-E, et al. Acrodermatitis Enteropathica: A Case Report. *Medicine* 2016; 95(20): e3553-e.
247. Lai J, Moxey A, Nowak G, et al. The efficacy of zinc supplementation in depression: Systematic review of randomised controlled trials. *Journal of Affective Disorders* 2012; 136(1): e31-e9.
248. Naguib YW, Saha S, Skeie JM, et al. Solubilized ubiquinol for preserving corneal function. *Biomaterials* 2021; 275: 120842.
249. Orlando P, Silvestri S, Galeazzi R, et al. Effect of ubiquinol supplementation on biochemical and oxidative stress indexes after intense exercise in young athletes. *Redox Rep* 2018; 23(1): 136-45.
250. Diaz-Castro J, Moreno-Fernandez J, Chirosa I, et al. Beneficial Effect of Ubiquinol on Hematological and Inflammatory Signaling during Exercise. *Nutrients* 2020; 12(2).
251. Garrido-Maraver J, Cordero MD, Oropesa-Avila M, et al. Clinical applications of coenzyme Q10. *Frontiers in bioscience (Landmark edition)* 2014; 19: 619-33.
252. Hargreaves IP, Mantle D. Coenzyme Q10 Supplementation in Fibrosis and Aging. *Adv Exp Med Biol* 2019; 1178: 103-12.
253. Sabbatinelli J, Orlando P, Galeazzi R, et al. Ubiquinol Ameliorates Endothelial Dysfunction in Subjects with Mild-to-Moderate Dyslipidemia: A Randomized Clinical Trial. *Nutrients* 2020; 12(4).
254. Lei L, Liu Y. Efficacy of coenzyme Q10 in patients with cardiac failure: a meta-analysis of clinical trials. *BMC Cardiovasc Disord* 2017; 17(1): 196.
255. Lee BJ, Tseng YF, Yen CH, et al. Effects of coenzyme Q10 supplementation (300 mg/day) on antioxidation and anti-inflammation in coronary artery disease patients during statins therapy: a randomized, placebo-controlled trial. *Nutrition journal* 2013; 12(1): 142.
256. Tiano L, Belardinelli R, Carnevali P, et al. Effect of coenzyme Q10 administration on endothelial function and extracellular superoxide dismutase in patients with ischaemic heart disease: a double-blind, randomized controlled study. *Eur Heart J* 2007; 28(18): 2249-55.
257. Handy DE, Loscalzo J. The role of glutathione peroxidase-1 in health and disease. *Free Radic Biol Med* 2022; 188: 146-61.
258. Lubos E, Loscalzo J, Handy DE. Glutathione peroxidase-1 in health and disease: from molecular mechanisms to therapeutic opportunities. *Antioxidants & redox signaling* 2011; 15(7): 1957-97.
259. Farag A, Abass W, Qassem H. Evaluation of the antioxidant and anti-inflammatory effect of sublingual glutathione on COPD patients. *J Med Life* 2023; 16(12): 1796-801.
260. Dalvi SM, Patil VW, Ramraje NN. The roles of glutathione, glutathione peroxidase, glutathione reductase and the carbonyl protein in pulmonary and extra pulmonary tuberculosis. *J Clin Diagn Res* 2012; 6(9): 1462-5.
261. Moran LJ, Grieger JA, Mishra GD, et al. The Association of a Mediterranean-Style Diet Pattern with Polycystic Ovary Syndrome Status in a Community Cohort Study. *Nutrients* 2015; 7(10): 8553-64.
262. Widmer RJ, Flammer AJ, Lerman LO, et al. The Mediterranean diet, its components, and cardiovascular disease. *Am J Med* 2015; 128(3): 229-38.
263. Di Tucci C, Di Feliciantonio M, Vena F, et al. Alpha lipoic acid in obstetrics and gynecology. *Gynecol Endocrinol* 2018; 34(9): 729-33.
264. Bast A, Haenen GR. Lipoic acid: a multifunctional antioxidant. *Biofactors* 2003; 17(1-4): 207-13.
265. Amini Khoozani A, Birch J, Bekhit AEA. Production, application and health effects of banana pulp and peel flour in the food industry. *J Food Sci Technol* 2019; 56(2): 548-59.
266. Bhuyan DJ, Alsherbiny MA, Perera S, et al. The Odyssey of Bioactive Compounds in Avocado (Persea americana) and Their Health Benefits. *Antioxidants (Basel)* 2019; 8(10).
267. Cao J, Schwichtenberg KA, Hanson NQ, et al. Incorporation and clearance of omega-3 fatty acids in erythrocyte membranes and plasma phospholipids. *Clin Chem* 2006; 52(12): 2265-72.
268. Jung UJ, Torrejon C, Tighe AP, et al. n-3 Fatty acids and cardiovascular disease: mechanisms underlying beneficial effects. *Am J Clin Nutr* 2008; 87(6): 2003S-9S.

269. Avallone R, Vitale G, Bertolotti M. Omega-3 Fatty Acids and Neurodegenerative Diseases: New Evidence in Clinical Trials. *International journal of molecular sciences* 2019; 20(17).
270. Ogłuszka M, Lipiński P, Starzyński RR. Effect of Omega-3 Fatty Acids on Telomeres-Are They the Elixir of Youth? *Nutrients* 2022; 14(18).
271. McEwen B, Morel-Kopp MC, Tofler G, et al. Effect of omega-3 fish oil on cardiovascular risk in diabetes. *Diabetes Educ* 2010; 36(4): 565-84.
272. McEwen BJ. The influence of diet and nutrients on platelet function. *Semin Thromb Hemost* 2014; 40(2): 214-26.
273. Sheikh O, Vande Hei AG, Battisha A, et al. Cardiovascular, electrophysiologic, and hematologic effects of omega-3 fatty acids beyond reducing hypertriglyceridemia: as it pertains to the recently published REDUCE-IT trial. *Cardiovascular diabetology* 2019; 18(1): 84.
274. Kiecolt-Glaser JK, Epel ES, Belury MA, et al. Omega-3 fatty acids, oxidative stress, and leukocyte telomere length: A randomized controlled trial. *Brain Behav Immun* 2013; 28: 16-24.
275. McEwen BJ, Morel-Kopp MC, Chen W, et al. Effects of omega-3 polyunsaturated fatty acids on platelet function in healthy subjects and subjects with cardiovascular disease. *Semin Thromb Hemost* 2013; 39(1): 25-32.
276. McEwen BJ, Morel-Kopp MC, Tofler GH, et al. The effect of omega-3 polyunsaturated fatty acids on fibrin and thrombin generation in healthy subjects and subjects with cardiovascular disease. *Semin Thromb Hemost* 2015; 41(3): 315-22.
277. McEwen BJ. Can omega-3 polyunsaturated fatty acids improve metabolic profile in polycystic ovary syndrome (PCOS)? *Advances in Integrative Medicine* 2017; 4(2): 82-3.
278. Bourre JM. Effects of nutrients (in food) on the structure and function of the nervous system: update on dietary requirements for brain. Part 2 : macronutrients. *The journal of nutrition, health & aging* 2006; 10(5): 386-99.
279. Østbye TK, Berge GM, Nilsson A, et al. The long-chain monounsaturated cetoleic acid improves the efficiency of the n-3 fatty acid metabolic pathway in Atlantic salmon and human HepG2 cells. *Br J Nutr* 2019; 122(7): 755-68.
280. Wakeman M. Equal effectiveness of omega-3 polyunsaturated fatty acids (n-3 PUFAs) from CET03® and fish oil in elevating the omega-3 index: A 12-week randomized placebo controlled parallel study. *International Journal of Scientific Research* 2024; 13(1).
281. Tobin D, Midtbø LK, Mildenberger J, et al. The effect of fish oil rich in cetoleic acid on the omega-3 index and skin quality. *Prostaglandins Leukot Essent Fatty Acids* 2024; 201: 102616.
282. Bhatt JK, Thomas S, Nanjan MJ. Resveratrol supplementation improves glycemic control in type 2 diabetes mellitus. *Nutr Res* 2012; 32(7): 537-41.
283. Kennedy DO, Wightman EL, Reay JL, et al. Effects of resveratrol on cerebral blood flow variables and cognitive performance in humans: a double-blind, placebo-controlled, crossover investigation. *Am J Clin Nutr* 2010; 91(6): 1590-7.
284. Breuss JM, Atanasov AG, Uhrin P. Resveratrol and Its Effects on the Vascular System. *International journal of molecular sciences* 2019; 20(7).
285. Tomé-Carneiro J, Larrosa M, Yáñez-Gascón MJ, et al. One-year supplementation with a grape extract containing resveratrol modulates inflammatory-related microRNAs and cytokines expression in peripheral blood mononuclear cells of type 2 diabetes and hypertensive patients with coronary artery disease. *Pharmacological research : the official journal of the Italian Pharmacological Society* 2013; 72: 69-82.
286. Zhou DD, Luo M, Huang SY, et al. Effects and Mechanisms of Resveratrol on Aging and Age-Related Diseases. *Oxidative medicine and cellular longevity* 2021; 2021: 9932218.
287. Huang H, Chen G, Liao D, et al. The effects of resveratrol intervention on risk markers of cardiovascular health in overweight and obese subjects: a pooled analysis of randomized controlled trials. *Obes Rev* 2016; 17(12): 1329-40.
288. Pistone G, Marino A, Leotta C, et al. Levocarnitine administration in elderly subjects with rapid muscle fatigue: effect on body composition, lipid profile and fatigue. *Drugs & aging* 2003; 20(10): 761-7.
289. Barnish M, Sheikh M, Scholey A. Nutrient Therapy for the Improvement of Fatigue Symptoms. *Nutrients* 2023; 15(9).
290. Durazzo A, Lucarini M, Nazhand A, et al. The Nutraceutical Value of Carnitine and Its Use in Dietary Supplements. *Molecules* 2020; 25(9).

291. Vermeulen RC, Scholte HR. Exploratory open label, randomized study of acetyl- and propionylcarnitine in chronic fatigue syndrome. *Psychosom Med* 2004; 66(2): 276-82.
292. Forbes SC, Cordingley DM, Cornish SM, et al. Effects of Creatine Supplementation on Brain Function and Health. *Nutrients* 2022; 14(5).
293. Forbes SC, Candow DG, Neto JHF, et al. Creatine supplementation and endurance performance: surges and sprints to win the race. *J Int Soc Sports Nutr* 2023; 20(1): 2204071.
294. Prokopidis K, Giannos P, Triantafyllidis KK, et al. Effects of creatine supplementation on memory in healthy individuals: a systematic review and meta-analysis of randomized controlled trials. *Nutrition reviews* 2023; 81(4): 416-27.
295. Gordji-Nejad A, Matusch A, Kleedörfer S, et al. Single dose creatine improves cognitive performance and induces changes in cerebral high energy phosphates during sleep deprivation. *Scientific reports* 2024; 14(1): 4937.
296. Dolan E, Gualano B, Rawson ES. Beyond muscle: the effects of creatine supplementation on brain creatine, cognitive processing, and traumatic brain injury. *Eur J Sport Sci* 2019; 19(1): 1-14.
297. McMorris T, Mielcarz G, Harris RC, et al. Creatine supplementation and cognitive performance in elderly individuals. *Neuropsychol Dev Cogn B Aging Neuropsychol Cogn* 2007; 14(5): 517-28.
298. Rawson ES, Venezia AC. Use of creatine in the elderly and evidence for effects on cognitive function in young and old. *Amino acids* 2011; 40(5): 1349-62.
299. Liu D, Chen Z. The regulatory effects of glutamine on illness and health. *Protein and peptide letters* 2011; 18(7): 658-62.
300. Meynial-Denis D. Glutamine metabolism in advanced age. *Nutrition reviews* 2016; 74(4): 225-36.
301. Coqueiro AY, Rogero MM, Tirapegui J. Glutamine as an Anti-Fatigue Amino Acid in Sports Nutrition. *Nutrients* 2019; 11(4).
302. Curi R, Lagranha CJ, Doi SQ, et al. Molecular mechanisms of glutamine action. *J Cell Physiol* 2005; 204(2): 392-401.
303. Cruzat V, Macedo Rogero M, Noel Keane K, et al. Glutamine: Metabolism and Immune Function, Supplementation and Clinical Translation. *Nutrients* 2018; 10(11).
304. Wang B, Wu G, Zhou Z, et al. Glutamine and intestinal barrier function. *Amino acids* 2015; 47(10): 2143-54.
305. Kim MH, Kim H. The Roles of Glutamine in the Intestine and Its Implication in Intestinal Diseases. *International journal of molecular sciences* 2017; 18(5).
306. Gleeson M. Dosing and efficacy of glutamine supplementation in human exercise and sport training. *J Nutr* 2008; 138(10): 2045s-9s.
307. Lardner AL. Neurobiological effects of the green tea constituent theanine and its potential role in the treatment of psychiatric and neurodegenerative disorders. *Nutr Neurosci* 2014; 17(4): 145-55.
308. Hidese S, Ogawa S, Ota M, et al. Effects of L-Theanine Administration on Stress-Related Symptoms and Cognitive Functions in Healthy Adults: A Randomized Controlled Trial. *Nutrients* 2019; 11(10).
309. Li MY, Liu HY, Wu DT, et al. L-Theanine: A Unique Functional Amino Acid in Tea (Camellia sinensis L.) With Multiple Health Benefits and Food Applications. *Front Nutr* 2022; 9: 853846.
310. Yoto A, Motoki M, Murao S, et al. Effects of L-theanine or caffeine intake on changes in blood pressure under physical and psychological stresses. *J Physiol Anthropol* 2012; 31(1): 28.
311. Hidese S, Ota M, Wakabayashi C, et al. Effects of chronic l-theanine administration in patients with major depressive disorder: an open-label study. *Acta Neuropsychiatr* 2017; 29(2): 72-9.
312. Kimura K, Ozeki M, Juneja LR, et al. L-Theanine reduces psychological and physiological stress responses. *Biol Psychol* 2007; 74(1): 39-45.
313. Chen S, Kang J, Zhu H, et al. L-Theanine and Immunity: A Review. *Molecules* 2023; 28(9).
314. Williams JL, Everett JM, D'Cunha NM, et al. The Effects of Green Tea Amino Acid L-Theanine Consumption on the Ability to Manage Stress and Anxiety Levels: a Systematic Review. *Plant Foods Hum Nutr* 2020; 75(1): 12-23.

315. Kim DU, Chung HC, Choi J, et al. Oral Intake of Low-Molecular-Weight Collagen Peptide Improves Hydration, Elasticity, and Wrinkling in Human Skin: A Randomized, Double-Blind, Placebo-Controlled Study. *Nutrients* 2018; 10(7).
316. Choi FD, Sung CT, Juhasz ML, et al. Oral Collagen Supplementation: A Systematic Review of Dermatological Applications. *J Drugs Dermatol* 2019; 18(1): 9-16.
317. de Miranda RB, Weimer P, Rossi RC. Effects of hydrolyzed collagen supplementation on skin aging: a systematic review and meta-analysis. *Int J Dermatol* 2021; 60(12): 1449-61.
318. Martínez-Puig D, Costa-Larrión E, Rubio-Rodríguez N, et al. Collagen Supplementation for Joint Health: The Link between Composition and Scientific Knowledge. *Nutrients* 2023; 15(6).
319. García-Coronado JM, Martínez-Olvera L, Elizondo-Omaña RE, et al. Effect of collagen supplementation on osteoarthritis symptoms: a meta-analysis of randomized placebo-controlled trials. *Int Orthop* 2019; 43(3): 531-8.
320. Lugo JP, Saiyed ZM, Lau FC, et al. Undenatured type II collagen (UC-II®) for joint support: a randomized, double-blind, placebo-controlled study in healthy volunteers. *J Int Soc Sports Nutr* 2013; 10(1): 48.
321. Kumar P, Bansal P, Rajnish RK, et al. Efficacy of undenatured collagen in knee osteoarthritis: review of the literature with limited meta-analysis. *Am J Transl Res* 2023; 15(9): 5545-55.
322. Crowley DC, Lau FC, Sharma P, et al. Safety and efficacy of undenatured type II collagen in the treatment of osteoarthritis of the knee: a clinical trial. *Int J Med Sci* 2009; 6(6): 312-21.
323. Lugo JP, Saiyed ZM, Lane NE. Efficacy and tolerability of an undenatured type II collagen supplement in modulating knee osteoarthritis symptoms: a multicenter randomized, double-blind, placebo-controlled study. *Nutrition journal* 2016; 15: 14.
324. Saiyed Z, Durkee S, Bowman J, et al. Efficacy of UC-II® undenatured type II collagen on knee joint function in healthy subjects: an exploratory post hoc analyses of a randomized double blind, placebo - controlled trial. *The FASEB Journal* 2021; 35(S1).
325. Schön C, Knaub K, Alt W, et al. UC-II Undenatured Type II Collagen for Knee Joint Flexibility: A Multicenter, Randomized, Double-Blind, Placebo-Controlled Clinical Study. *J Integr Complement Med* 2022; 28(6): 540-8.
326. D'Amico D, Andreux PA, Valdés P, et al. Impact of the Natural Compound Urolithin A on Health, Disease, and Aging. *Trends Mol Med* 2021; 27(7): 687-99.
327. Ryu D, Mouchiroud L, Andreux PA, et al. Urolithin A induces mitophagy and prolongs lifespan in C. elegans and increases muscle function in rodents. *Nat Med* 2016; 22(8): 879-88.
328. D'Amico D, Olmer M, Fouassier AM, et al. Urolithin A improves mitochondrial health, reduces cartilage degeneration, and alleviates pain in osteoarthritis. *Aging Cell* 2022; 21(8): e13662.
329. Craig WJ. Health-promoting properties of common herbs. *Am J Clin Nutr* 1999; 70(3 Suppl): 491S-9S.
330. Vickers A, Zollman C. ABC of complementary medicine: herbal medicine. *BMJ* 1999; 319(7216): 1050-3.
331. Krivoy N, Pavlotzky E, Chrubasik S, et al. Effect of salicis cortex extract on human platelet aggregation. *Planta medica* 2001; 67(3): 209-12.
332. Miraj S, Rafieian K, Kiani S. Melissa officinalis L: A Review Study With an Antioxidant Prospective. *J Evid Based Complementary Altern Med* 2017; 22(3): 385-94.
333. Szczuka D, Nowak A, Zakłos-Szyda M, et al. American Ginseng (Panax quinquefolium L.) as a Source of Bioactive Phytochemicals with Pro-Health Properties. *Nutrients* 2019; 11(5).
334. White DJ, Camfield DA, Ossoukhova A, et al. Effects of Panax quinquefolius (American ginseng) on the steady state visually evoked potential during cognitive performance. *Human psychopharmacology* 2020; 35(6): 1-6.
335. Ali N, Ali Shah SW, Shah I, et al. Anthelmintic and relaxant activities of Verbascum Thapsus Mullein. *BMC Complement Altern Med* 2012; 12: 29.
336. Och A, Och M, Nowak R, et al. Berberine, a Herbal Metabolite in the Metabolic Syndrome: The Risk Factors, Course, and Consequences of the Disease. *Molecules* 2022; 27(4).
337. Pérez-Rubio KG, González-Ortiz M, Martínez-Abundis E, et al. Effect of berberine administration on metabolic syndrome, insulin sensitivity, and insulin secretion. *Metab Syndr Relat Disord* 2013; 11(5): 366-9.

338. Nemetchek MD, Stierle AA, Stierle DB, et al. The Ayurvedic plant Bacopa monnieri inhibits inflammatory pathways in the brain. *Journal of ethnopharmacology* 2017; 197: 92-100.
339. Amsterdam JD, Shults J, Soeller I, et al. Chamomile (Matricaria recutita) may provide antidepressant activity in anxious, depressed humans: an exploratory study. *Altern Ther Health Med* 2012; 18(5): 44-9.
340. Brenyo A, Aktas MK. Review of complementary and alternative medical treatment of arrhythmias. *Am J Cardiol* 2014; 113(5): 897-903.
341. Kunnumakkara AB, Bordoloi D, Padmavathi G, et al. Curcumin, the golden nutraceutical: multitargeting for multiple chronic diseases. *British journal of pharmacology* 2017; 174(11): 1325-48.
342. Hosseini A, Hosseinzadeh H. Antidotal or protective effects of Curcuma longa (turmeric) and its active ingredient, curcumin, against natural and chemical toxicities: A review. *Biomed Pharmacother* 2018; 99: 411-21.
343. Choudhary B, Shetty A, Langade DG. Efficacy of Ashwagandha (Withania somnifera [L.] Dunal) in improving cardiorespiratory endurance in healthy athletic adults. *Ayu* 2015; 36(1): 63-8.
344. Choudhary D, Bhattacharyya S, Bose S. Efficacy and Safety of Ashwagandha (Withania somnifera (L.) Dunal) Root Extract in Improving Memory and Cognitive Functions. *Journal of dietary supplements* 2017; 14(6): 599-612.
345. Punukollu RS, Chadalawada AK, Siddabattuni K, et al. A blend of Withania somnifera (L.) Dunal root and Abelmoschus esculentus (L.) Moench fruit extracts relieves constipation and improves bowel function: A proof-of-concept clinical investigation. *Journal of ethnopharmacology* 2024; 318(Pt B): 116997.
346. Sarris J, McIntyre E, Camfield DA. Plant-based medicines for anxiety disorders, part 2: a review of clinical studies with supporting preclinical evidence. *CNS drugs* 2013; 27(4): 301-19.
347. Singh G, Dixit I, Kalman D, et al. A Novel Herbal Composition Alleviates Functional Constipation, Reduces Gastrointestinal Transit Time, and Improves Bowel Function in Adults: A Double-Blind, Randomized Clinical Study. *J Am Nutr Assoc* 2024; 43(6): 553-66.
348. Belwal T, Bisht A, Devkota HP, et al. Phytopharmacology and Clinical Updates of Berberis Species Against Diabetes and Other Metabolic Diseases. *Front Pharmacol* 2020; 11: 41.
349. Zhang Y, Li X, Zou D, et al. Treatment of type 2 diabetes and dyslipidemia with the natural plant alkaloid berberine. *J Clin Endocrinol Metab* 2008; 93(7): 2559-65.
350. Cao C, Su M. Effects of berberine on glucose-lipid metabolism, inflammatory factors and insulin resistance in patients with metabolic syndrome. *Experimental and therapeutic medicine* 2019; 17(4): 3009-14.
351. Kong W, Wei J, Abidi P, et al. Berberine is a novel cholesterol-lowering drug working through a unique mechanism distinct from statins. *Nat Med* 2004; 10(12): 1344-51.
352. Russo A, Borrelli F. Bacopa monniera, a reputed nootropic plant: an overview. *Phytomedicine* 2005; 12(4): 305-17.
353. Pase MP, Kean J, Sarris J, et al. The cognitive-enhancing effects of Bacopa monnieri: a systematic review of randomized, controlled human clinical trials. *J Altern Complement Med* 2012; 18(7): 647-52.
354. Stough C, Downey LA, Lloyd J, et al. Examining the nootropic effects of a special extract of Bacopa monniera on human cognitive functioning: 90 day double-blind placebo-controlled randomized trial. *Phytother Res* 2008; 22(12): 1629-34.
355. Calabrese C, Gregory WL, Leo M, et al. Effects of a standardized Bacopa monnieri extract on cognitive performance, anxiety, and depression in the elderly: a randomized, double-blind, placebo-controlled trial. *J Altern Complement Med* 2008; 14(6): 707-13.
356. Kongkeaw C, Dilokthornsakul P, Thanarangsarit P, et al. Meta-analysis of randomized controlled trials on cognitive effects of Bacopa monnieri extract. *Journal of ethnopharmacology* 2014; 151(1): 528-35.
357. Stough C, Lloyd J, Clarke J, et al. The chronic effects of an extract of Bacopa monniera (Brahmi) on cognitive function in healthy human subjects. *Psychopharmacology (Berl)* 2001; 156(4): 481-4.
358. Singh N, Garg M, Prajapati P, et al. Adaptogenic property of Asparagus racemosus: Future trends and prospects. *Heliyon* 2023; 9(4): e14932.

359. Zahid H, Rizwani GH, Ishaqe S. Phytopharmacological Review on Vitex agnus-castus: A Potential Medicinal Plant. *Chinese Herbal Medicines* 2016; 8(1): 24-9.
360. Zamani M, Neghab N, Torabian S. Therapeutic effect of Vitex agnus castus in patients with premenstrual syndrome. *Acta Med Iran* 2012; 50(2): 101-6.
361. Rafieian-Kopaei M, Movahedi M. Systematic Review of Premenstrual, Postmenstrual and Infertility Disorders of Vitex Agnus Castus. *Electron Physician* 2017; 9(1): 3685-9.
362. Hossein-Rashidi B, Nemati M. Effects of Vitex agnus-castus extract on the secretory function of pituitary-gonadal axis and pregnancy rate in patients with premature ovarian aging (POA). *Journal of Herbal Medicine* 2017; 10: 24-30.
363. Carmichael AR. Can Vitex Agnus Castus be Used for the Treatment of Mastalgia? What is the Current Evidence? *Evidence-based complementary and alternative medicine : eCAM* 2008; 5(3): 247-50.
364. Wuttke W, Jarry H, Christoffel V, et al. Chaste tree (Vitex agnus-castus)--pharmacology and clinical indications. *Phytomedicine* 2003; 10(4): 348-57.
365. Stephens L, Whitehouse J, Polley M. Western herbal medicine, epigenetics, and endometriosis. *J Altern Complement Med* 2013; 19(11): 853-9.
366. Low Dog T. Conventional and alternative treatments for endometriosis. *Altern Ther Health Med* 2001; 7(6): 50-6; quiz 7.
367. He Z, Chen R, Zhou Y, et al. Treatment for premenstrual syndrome with Vitex agnus castus: A prospective, randomized, multi-center placebo controlled study in China. *Maturitas* 2009; 63(1): 99-103.
368. Yi L, Liang Y, Wu H, et al. The analysis of Radix Angelicae Sinensis (Danggui). *Journal of Chromatography A* 2009; 1216(11): 1991-2001.
369. Page RL, 2nd, Lawrence JD. Potentiation of warfarin by dong quai. *Pharmacotherapy* 1999; 19(7): 870-6.
370. Sharifi-Rad M, Mnayer D, Morais-Braga MFB, et al. Echinacea plants as antioxidant and antibacterial agents: From traditional medicine to biotechnological applications. *Phytother Res* 2018; 32(9): 1653-63.
371. Catanzaro M, Corsini E, Rosini M, et al. Immunomodulators Inspired by Nature: A Review on Curcumin and Echinacea. *Molecules (Basel, Switzerland)* 2018; 23(11): 2778.
372. Hudson JB. Applications of the phytomedicine Echinacea purpurea (Purple Coneflower) in infectious diseases. *Journal of biomedicine & biotechnology* 2012; 2012: 769896-.
373. Ross SM. Echinacea purpurea: A Proprietary Extract of Echinacea purpurea Is Shown to be Safe and Effective in the Prevention of the Common Cold. *Holist Nurs Pract* 2016; 30(1): 54-7.
374. Heinonen T, Gaus W. Cross matching observations on toxicological and clinical data for the assessment of tolerability and safety of Ginkgo biloba leaf extract. *Toxicology* 2015; 327C: 95-115.
375. Kudolo GB, Dorsey S, Blodgett J. Effect of the ingestion of Ginkgo biloba extract on platelet aggregation and urinary prostanoid excretion in healthy and Type 2 diabetic subjects. *Thromb Res* 2002; 108(2-3): 151-60.
376. Kargozar R, Azizi H, Salari R. A review of effective herbal medicines in controlling menopausal symptoms. *Electron Physician* 2017; 9(11): 5826-33.
377. Gardner CD, Zehnder JL, Rigby AJ, et al. Effect of Ginkgo biloba (EGb 761) and aspirin on platelet aggregation and platelet function analysis among older adults at risk of cardiovascular disease: a randomized clinical trial. *Blood Coagul Fibrinolysis* 2007; 18(8): 787-93.
378. Amieva H, Meillon C, Helmer C, et al. Ginkgo biloba extract and long-term cognitive decline: a 20-year follow-up population-based study. *PLoS One* 2013; 8(1): e52755.
379. Jung F, Mrowietz C, Kiesewetter H, et al. Effect of Ginkgo biloba on fluidity of blood and peripheral microcirculation in volunteers. *Arzneimittelforschung* 1990; 40(5): 589-93.
380. Lamant V, Mauco G, Braquet P, et al. Inhibition of the metabolism of platelet activating factor (PAF-acether) by three specific antagonists from Ginkgo biloba. *Biochem Pharmacol* 1987; 36(17): 2749-52.
381. Chen CL, Tsai WH, Chen CJ, et al. Centella asiatica extract protects against amyloid β(1-40)-induced neurotoxicity in neuronal cells by activating the antioxidative defence system. *J Tradit Complement Med* 2016; 6(4): 362-9.
382. Gohil KJ, Patel JA, Gajjar AK. Pharmacological Review on Centella asiatica: A Potential Herbal Cure-all. *Indian J Pharm Sci* 2010; 72(5): 546-56.

383. Torbati FA, Ramezani M, Dehghan R, et al. Ethnobotany, Phytochemistry and Pharmacological Features of Centella asiatica: A Comprehensive Review. *Adv Exp Med Biol* 2021; 1308: 451-99.
384. Brinkhaus B, Lindner M, Schuppan D, et al. Chemical, pharmacological and clinical profile of the East Asian medical plant Centella asiatica. *Phytomedicine* 2000; 7(5): 427-48.
385. Wattanathorn J, Mator L, Muchimapura S, et al. Positive modulation of cognition and mood in the healthy elderly volunteer following the administration of Centella asiatica. *Journal of ethnopharmacology* 2008; 116(2): 325-32.
386. Subathra M, Shila S, Devi MA, et al. Emerging role of Centella asiatica in improving age-related neurological antioxidant status. *Exp Gerontol* 2005; 40(8-9): 707-15.
387. Jana U, Sur TK, Maity LN, et al. A clinical study on the management of generalized anxiety disorder with Centella asiatica. *Nepal Med Coll J* 2010; 12(1): 8-11.
388. Bradwejn J, Zhou Y, Koszycki D, et al. A double-blind, placebo-controlled study on the effects of Gotu Kola (Centella asiatica) on acoustic startle response in healthy subjects. *J Clin Psychopharmacol* 2000; 20(6): 680-4.
389. Lee CH, Kim JH. A review on the medicinal potentials of ginseng and ginsenosides on cardiovascular diseases. *Journal of ginseng research* 2014; 38(3): 161-6.
390. Jin Y, Cui R, Zhao L, et al. Mechanisms of Panax ginseng action as an antidepressant. *Cell Prolif* 2019; 52(6): e12696.
391. Kim HG, Cho JH, Yoo SR, et al. Antifatigue effects of Panax ginseng C.A. Meyer: a randomised, double-blind, placebo-controlled trial. *PLoS One* 2013; 8(4): e61271.
392. Scholey A, Ossoukhova A, Owen L, et al. Effects of American ginseng (Panax quinquefolius) on neurocognitive function: an acute, randomised, double-blind, placebo-controlled, crossover study. *Psychopharmacology (Berl)* 2010; 212(3): 345-56.
393. Reay JL, Kennedy DO, Scholey AB. Single doses of Panax ginseng (G115) reduce blood glucose levels and improve cognitive performance during sustained mental activity. *J Psychopharmacol* 2005; 19(4): 357-65.
394. Lau AJ, Toh DF, Chua TK, et al. Antiplatelet and anticoagulant effects of Panax notoginseng: comparison of raw and steamed Panax notoginseng with Panax ginseng and Panax quinquefolium. *Journal of ethnopharmacology* 2009; 125(3): 380-6.
395. Kennedy DO, Wake G, Savelev S, et al. Modulation of mood and cognitive performance following acute administration of single doses of Melissa officinalis (Lemon balm) with human CNS nicotinic and muscarinic receptor-binding properties. *Neuropsychopharmacology* 2003; 28(10): 1871-81.
396. Shakeri A, Sahebkar A, Javadi B. Melissa officinalis L. - A review of its traditional uses, phytochemistry and pharmacology. *Journal of ethnopharmacology* 2016; 188: 204-28.
397. Scholey A, Gibbs A, Neale C, et al. Anti-stress effects of lemon balm-containing foods. *Nutrients* 2014; 6(11): 4805-21.
398. Kennedy DO, Little W, Scholey AB. Attenuation of laboratory-induced stress in humans after acute administration of Melissa officinalis (Lemon Balm). *Psychosom Med* 2004; 66(4): 607-13.
399. Flora K, Hahn M, Rosen H, et al. Milk thistle (Silybum marianum) for the therapy of liver disease. *Am J Gastroenterol* 1998; 93(2): 139-43.
400. Abenavoli L, Izzo AA, Milić N, et al. Milk thistle (Silybum marianum): A concise overview on its chemistry, pharmacological, and nutraceutical uses in liver diseases. *Phytother Res* 2018; 32(11): 2202-13.
401. Abenavoli L, Capasso R, Milic N, et al. Milk thistle in liver diseases: past, present, future. *Phytother Res* 2010; 24(10): 1423-32.
402. Roy A, Shrivastava SL, Mandal SM. Functional properties of Okra Abelmoschus esculentus L.(Moench): traditional claims and scientific evidences. *Plant science today* 2014; 1(3): 121-30.
403. Bahari H, Shahraki Jazinaki M, Rahnama I, et al. The cardiometabolic benefits of okra-based treatment in prediabetes and diabetes: a systematic review and meta-analysis of randomized controlled trials. *Front Nutr* 2024; 11: 1454286.
404. Dehghan Shahreza F. Hibiscus esculentus and diabetes mellitus. *J Nephropharmacol* 2016; 5(2): 104-5.
405. Esmaeilzadeh D, Razavi BM, Hosseinzadeh H. Effect of Abelmoschus esculentus (okra) on metabolic syndrome: A review. *Phytother Res* 2020; 34(9): 2192-202.

406. Miroddi M, Calapai G, Navarra M, et al. Passiflora incarnata L.: ethnopharmacology, clinical application, safety and evaluation of clinical trials. *Journal of ethnopharmacology* 2013; 150(3): 791-804.
407. Janda K, Wojtkowska K, Jakubczyk K, et al. Passiflora incarnata in Neuropsychiatric Disorders-A Systematic Review. *Nutrients* 2020; 12(12).
408. Modabbernia A, Akhondzadeh S. Saffron, passionflower, valerian and sage for mental health. *The Psychiatric clinics of North America* 2013; 36(1): 85-91.
409. Sarris J. Herbal medicines in the treatment of psychiatric disorders: 10-year updated review. *Phytother Res* 2018; 32(7): 1147-62.
410. Sarris J, Panossian A, Schweitzer I, et al. Herbal medicine for depression, anxiety and insomnia: a review of psychopharmacology and clinical evidence. *European neuropsychopharmacology : the journal of the European College of Neuropsychopharmacology* 2011; 21(12): 841-60.
411. Kim M, Lim H-S, Lee H-H, et al. Role Identification of Passiflora Incarnata Linnaeus: A Mini Review. *Journal of menopausal medicine* 2017; 23(3): 156-9.
412. Panossian A, Wikman G, Sarris J. Rosenroot (Rhodiola rosea): traditional use, chemical composition, pharmacology and clinical efficacy. *Phytomedicine* 2010; 17(7): 481-93.
413. Perfumi M, Mattioli L. Adaptogenic and central nervous system effects of single doses of 3% rosavin and 1% salidroside Rhodiola rosea L. extract in mice. *Phytother Res* 2007; 21(1): 37-43.
414. Amsterdam JD, Panossian AG. Rhodiola rosea L. as a putative botanical antidepressant. *Phytomedicine* 2016; 23(7): 770-83.
415. Nabavi SF, Braidy N, Orhan IE, et al. Rhodiola rosea L. and Alzheimer's Disease: From Farm to Pharmacy. *Phytother Res* 2016; 30(4): 532-9.
416. Olsson EM, von Schéele B, Panossian AG. A randomised, double-blind, placebo-controlled, parallel-group study of the standardised extract shr-5 of the roots of Rhodiola rosea in the treatment of subjects with stress-related fatigue. *Planta medica* 2009; 75(2): 105-12.
417. Darbinyan V, Aslanyan G, Amroyan E, et al. Clinical trial of Rhodiola rosea L. extract SHR-5 in the treatment of mild to moderate depression. *Nord J Psychiatry* 2007; 61(5): 343-8.
418. Dwyer AV, Whitten DL, Hawrelak JA. Herbal medicines, other than St. John's Wort, in the treatment of depression: a systematic review. *Altern Med Rev* 2011; 16(1): 40-9.
419. Toth B, Hegyi P, Lantos T, et al. The Efficacy of Saffron in the Treatment of Mild to Moderate Depression: A Meta-analysis. *Planta medica* 2019; 85(1): 24-31.
420. Dai L, Chen L, Wang W. Safety and Efficacy of Saffron (Crocus sativus L.) for Treating Mild to Moderate Depression: A Systematic Review and Meta-analysis. *The Journal of nervous and mental disease* 2020; 208(4): 269-76.
421. Leone S, Recinella L, Chiavaroli A, et al. Phytotherapic use of the Crocus sativus L. (Saffron) and its potential applications: A brief overview. *Phytother Res* 2018; 32(12): 2364-75.
422. Lopresti AL, Drummond PD. Saffron (Crocus sativus) for depression: a systematic review of clinical studies and examination of underlying antidepressant mechanisms of action. *Human psychopharmacology* 2014; 29(6): 517-27.
423. Hausenblas HA, Saha D, Dubyak PJ, et al. Saffron (Crocus sativus L.) and major depressive disorder: a meta-analysis of randomized clinical trials. *Journal of integrative medicine* 2013; 11(6): 377-83.
424. Lopresti AL, Smith SJ, Marx W, et al. An Examination into the Effects of a Saffron Extract (Affron) on Mood and General Wellbeing in Adults Experiencing Low Mood: A Randomized, Double-Blind, Placebo-Controlled Trial. *J Nutr* 2025; 155(7): 2300-11.
425. Lopresti AL, Smith SJ, Metse AP, et al. Effects of saffron on sleep quality in healthy adults with self-reported poor sleep: a randomized, double-blind, placebo-controlled trial. *J Clin Sleep Med* 2020; 16(6): 937-47.
426. Munirah MP, Norhayati MN, Noraini M. Crocus Sativus for Insomnia: A Systematic Review and Meta-Analysis. *International journal of environmental research and public health* 2022; 19(18).
427. Moshiri M, Vahabzadeh M, Hosseinzadeh H. Clinical Applications of Saffron (Crocus sativus) and its Constituents: A Review. *Drug research* 2015; 65(6): 287-95.
428. Goyal RK, Singh J, Lal H. Asparagus racemosus--an update. *Indian J Med Sci* 2003; 57(9): 408-14.

429. Dalvi SS, Nadkarni PM, Gupta KC. Effect of Asparagus racemosus (Shatavari) on gastric emptying time in normal healthy volunteers. *J Postgrad Med* 1990; 36(2): 91-4.
430. Kohli D, Champawat PS, Mudgal VD. Asparagus (Asparagus racemosus L.) roots: nutritional profile, medicinal profile, preservation, and value addition. *J Sci Food Agric* 2023; 103(5): 2239-50.
431. Singh R. Asparagus racemosus: a review on its phytochemical and therapeutic potential. *Natural product research* 2016; 30(17): 1896-908.
432. O'Leary MF, Jackman SR, Sabou VR, et al. Shatavari Supplementation in Postmenopausal Women Improves Handgrip Strength and Increases Vastus lateralis Myosin Regulatory Light Chain Phosphorylation but Does Not Alter Markers of Bone Turnover. *Nutrients* 2021; 13(12).
433. O'Leary MF, Jackman SR, Bowtell JL. Shatavari supplementation in postmenopausal women alters the skeletal muscle proteome and pathways involved in training adaptation. *Eur J Nutr* 2024; 63(3): 869-79.
434. Kocaadam B, Sanlier N. Curcumin, an active component of turmeric (Curcuma longa), and its effects on health. *Crit Rev Food Sci Nutr* 2017; 57(13): 2889-95.
435. Rezzani R, Franco C, Rodella LF. Curcumin as a Therapeutic Strategy in Liver Diseases. *Nutrients* 2019; 11(10).
436. Campbell MS, Carlini NA, Fleenor BS. Influence of curcumin on performance and post-exercise recovery. *Crit Rev Food Sci Nutr* 2020: 1-11.
437. Sun J, Chen F, Braun C, et al. Role of curcumin in the management of pathological pain. *Phytomedicine* 2018; 48: 129-40.
438. Lopez-Malo D, Villaron-Casares CA, Alarcon-Jimenez J, et al. Curcumin as a Therapeutic Option in Retinal Diseases. *Antioxidants (Basel)* 2020; 9(1).
439. Chainoglou E, Hadjipavlou-Litina D. Curcumin in Health and Diseases: Alzheimer's Disease and Curcumin Analogues, Derivatives, and Hybrids. *International journal of molecular sciences* 2020; 21(6).
440. Slika L, Patra D. Traditional Uses, Therapeutic Effects and Recent Advances of Curcumin: A Mini-Review. *Mini Rev Med Chem* 2020.
441. Anonymous. Curcuma longa (turmeric). Monograph. *Altern Med Rev* 2001; 6 Suppl: S62-6.
442. Vaughn AR, Branum A, Sivamani RK. Effects of Turmeric (Curcuma longa) on Skin Health: A Systematic Review of the Clinical Evidence. *Phytother Res* 2016; 30(8): 1243-64.

NMN at a glance

Name	β-Nicotinamide Mononucleotide[105]		
Chemical formula	$C_{11}H_{15}N_2O_8P$[105]		
CAS number	1094-61-7[42,105]	**Molecular Weight**	334.22 g/mol[105]
Functions from various preclinical trials	increases NAD^+ levels,[40-46] increases cellular energy,[47] improve cellular glucose metabolism,[40] improves insulin action[46] and sensitivity,[46] Improves cellular lipid metabolism,[40] improves endothelial function,[50] protects the heart from ischaemia/reperfusion injury,[45] cardioprotective,[45] reduces age-related arterial stiffness,[50] improves endothelial function,[50] neuroprotection,[42,43] activates SIRT1,[42,50] stimulates autophagy,[45] anti-inflammatory,[41,42,48] antioxidant,[42,43] improves cell viability[41]		
Human Clinical Trials	• increases intracellular NAD^+ levels[98,101] • enhances NAD levels[39,97,108-113] • enhances muscle insulin signalling[110] • improves muscle insulin sensitivity[110] • improves arterial stiffness[114] • enhances muscle NAD^+ turnover[110] • decreases postprandial hyperinsulinaemia[101] • decreases total cholesterol[112] • decreases LDL cholesterol[112] • decreases apolipoprotein B levels[112] • decreases diastolic blood pressure[112] • improves motor function[115] • improves walking speed[109,115] • increases walking distance[108,111] • enhances aerobic capacity[116] • potentially improves maximal voluntary muscle strength[112] • shows potential in reducing body weight[112] • improved sleep quality[109] • improves longevity[111] • improves health-related quality of life[108,111]		
Daily dosage range	100 mg,[119] 125 mg,[101] 250 mg, [39,101,109,110,114,115,119] 300 mg,[108,111,116] 500 mg,[119] 600 mg,[108,111,116] 900 mg,[108,111] 1,000 mg,[112,113] 1,200 mg,[116] 1,250 mg,[120] 2,000 mg.[112,113]		
For information purposes only. Not a substitute for medical advice. If symptoms persist, talk to a health professional. Always read the label. Follow the directions for use.			

Notes

Made in the USA
Monee, IL
04 November 2026

67382352R00079